W9-DJI-633

GOLFERS
TAKE CARE
of
YOUR
BACK

SUSAN M. CARPENTER, P.T.
FLORENCE P. KENDALL, P.T.

ILLUSTRATIONS BY JOHN MARSHALL

Thistle Ridge Press
332 Bunn Hill Road
Vestal, New York 13850

Notice to the Reader: The suggestions in this book are not meant to be a substitute for the advice of a physician. If you know that you have a specific medical problem or if you have concern about doing moderate exercises, consult your physician before trying the tests, exercises, or suggestions in this book.

Illustrations by John Marshall
Cover Design by Dina Good
Editing, Page Design and Prepress Production by Karen Bernardo

©Thistle Ridge Press, 1995
All rights reserved.

Thistle Ridge Press, 332 Bunn Hill Road, Vestal, New York 13850. Printed and bound in the United States of America. All rights reserved under International and Pan-American Copyright Convention. No part of this book, including illustrations, may be reproduced in any manner whatsoever, including photocopying, electronic or mechanical transmission or storage, without prior written permission from the publisher, except by reviewers who may quote brief passages to be printed in a magazine or newspaper.

First Printing 1995
00 99   5 4

Publisher's Cataloguing-in-Publication Data

Carpenter, Susan M., and Kendall, Florence P.
        Golfers, take care of your back
        Includes index
        1. Golf   2. Back pain   3. Exercise   4. Posture
ISBN 0-9637535-0-9
                        Library of Congress Catalog Card Number 94-90020

Dedicated
to
my parents
Charlotte and Donald McKinley
who taught me about the fun, joy, and friendship
the game of golf offers

Susan M. Carpenter

ACKNOWLEDGMENTS

A special thanks to the following people:

Dr. Charles Carpenter, who believed in the concept of "Back School" and encouraged the idea of producing this book; Don and Bob Carpenter who kept life full of fun and activity while the book was in progress.

Alex Alexander, chairman of the B.C. Open, En-Joie Golf Course, Endicott, New York, who recognized the need, and provided the opportunity, to present an educational seminar about the management of back pain to the PGA players. The B.C. Open has the distinction of being the first tournament on the PGA tour to have offered such a program.

Gina Kucharek, the first assistant for the back seminar presented at the B.C. Open; also, as office manager of Orthopedic Associates, she has been instrumental in supporting this project. Dr. Arthur White and Mrs. Lynne White for their instruction in the "Back School" approach. Tammy Thomas, for her help with the computer. Sandie and Gary Gardner, long-time friends who listened to ideas and gave "clear-thinking advice" on the concept of this book. Elizabeth, Kathryn, and Andrea Kerr, for their enthusiastic encouragement. Al Weiner, who saw that this book could be a reality. Dennis Molter, a great athlete and outdoorsman, who helped detail many aspects of the game. Robert Everett, for his dedication and interest in sports, and Richard Donovan who shared his experience as a publisher and collector of golf books.

Special thanks to the readers of this manuscript for their helpful suggestions: Dr. Tom and Gail Lewis; Dr. Larry Schenk; Dr. Maura Santangelo; Dr. Kamlesh Desai; Clem Poteran; James Caruso; David Lashier; Randy Metzler; Joyce Roser; Jan Kleiman; Lea Alvy; Ginny Nolan, P.T.; Chris Hoke, P.T.; Melanie Hewitt, P.T.; George McLean, P.T.; Ann Douglas; John Dunigan; Dr. Michael McClure; Kathleen McKinley; Scott Banks, Ph.D.; Dick and Lynda Kroboth; Diane Simmons; Judith Browne; Adrienne Parry, P.T.; Bill Burtis; William Rincker; Peter Hankin; Ralph Simpson, P.T., A.T.C.; Joan Wittan; Louis (Tuck) and Florence K. Tyler; and Charles and Susan Nolte.

ABOUT THE AUTHORS

Taking lessons from a golf professional is the best way to understand the game of golf and to learn the fundamentals of the golf swing.

Taking lessons from a health professional is the best way to learn how the body works in response to the game of golf.

Susan McKinley Carpenter has managed a physical therapy program called "The Back Works" for twenty years. This program teaches people to analyze how they perform their daily activities. It emphasizes good body mechanics, posture, corrective exercises, and prevention of the recurrence of back problems. Many of her patients have been recreational golfers.

When a professional golfer came to her as a patient, his shoulder muscles were very tight. He said he spent half a season limbering up. After teaching him how to stretch his muscles properly, he was able to *begin* his season with his "mid-season" swing.

For several years, at the B. C. Open, Susan conducted a class for professional golfers on the management of low back pain.

It became apparent that both recreational and professional golfers need information about the care of their backs, and the idea of writing a book became a challenge. In the hope of offering a clear, concise, and accurate presentation, Susan sought assistance from a long-time friend and author, Florence Kendall.

Florence Peterson Kendall is a world-renowned physical therapist, lecturer, and educator. The work of Florence and her late husband, Henry, in the field of muscle testing, posture, and pain serve as the foundation for physical therapists in the treatment and education of their patients. She is dedicated to excellence, and, as an author, precise in her words. Through her warmth, generosity, and concern, she has devoted herself to doing all she can to educate physical therapists in the basic knowledge of muscle function.

Many of the fundamentals of her teachings are now being made available to you, a golfer. Highly technical, accurate information is being presented in non-technical language so that you can apply this information to your golf game and daily activities.

Florence is co-author of *Posture and Pain* and four editions of *MUSCLES, Testing and Function. MUSCLES* has been published in eight foreign languages. She has served as Consultant to the Surgeon General, U.S. Army.

Her knowledge of anatomy and muscle function has led her to buck mainstream ideas on "fitness" and dispel many misconceptions about the function of abdominal muscles. Watch for her publication on the *Politics of Polio,* a fascinating account of how she and her husband had to deal with politics in the treatment of poliomyelitis.

TABLE OF CONTENTS

FOREWORDS BY GOLFERS*

"This book is great for the average golfer because all of us at one time or another will experience some form of back pain, usually from some kind of athletic activity. This book is very concise and gives you simple remedies for a variety of aches and pains."

Wayne Levi
P.G.A. Tour Professional

"The older I get, the more I realize the importance of a back maintenance program. The golf swing places such strain on the back. No matter how good your swing is, you need to care for your back. The authors understand and give many good ideas to keep a healthy back. Remember to warm up before getting to the driving range."

Bobby Clampett
P.G.A. Tour Professional

"This book provides an insightful, instructional, and intelligently compiled resource not only for the golfer's use, but also as an excellent primer for the clinician interested in treating 'the golfer's back'."

Ralph Simpson, P.T., A.T.C.

"I have felt privileged to review this book. The concepts are presented so clearly and logically that the aging golfer will immediately recognize that there is hope to reclaim his youth in the second nine of life. Never walk up to the first tee without doing some of the loosening-up routine in this book. Then, even if chronologically quite old, you can swing back farther and reach really high in the back-swing, bringing on a better turn and giving you a good swing-through to send the ball in the desired direction. One will seem younger through better posture and feel better from reawakening muscles and joints by stretching. If improved golf is the by-product, well, HOT-DOG!"

Rolla D. Campbell Jr., M.D.
Orthopaedic Surgeon
Author of book-in-progress, *Old Back, New Golf,* and, with Dan Colvin, P.G.A. Professional, a video, *Swing for a Lifetime.* Coordinator of the former Senior Golfer's Fitness and Imagery Swing Clinic in Jupiter, Florida

* Continued on back cover

GOLFERS
TAKE CARE
— *of* —
YOUR
BACK

INTRODUCTION

Golfers are a unique group of people. They are so dedicated to golf and so highly motivated that when they develop a problem which interferes with their game they will do "whatever it takes" to get better. This book aims to help them do just that.

The need for this book is based on the fact that golfers who understand the mechanics of golf often do not understand the mechanics of the body and how it responds to the demands of the game. Our challenge has been to take these two complex subjects and bring them together in a simple, uncomplicated form.

Of all the problems that trouble the golfer, low back pain appears to be the most common. But low back pain is not a simple problem, isolated and unrelated to the rest of the body. Restricted or excessive motion in other parts of the spine or other joints can give rise to low back problems.

Although there are many causes of back pain, the vast majority are muscular or mechanical in nature. Most of these cases can be helped by understanding how the back works and how muscle tightness or weakness and poor postural positions contribute to the problem.

Chapter One provides a quick lesson in the anatomy of the back as related to movements of the back and positions of the body during the golf swing.

Chapter Two covers easy walking and warm-up exercises to help you get in peak condition because players should get fit to play golf, not play golf to get fit.

Chapter Three, which covers self-tests and exercises, can help you determine the neces-sary and appropriate exercises to maintain or improve your ability to play golf.

Because the subject of abdominal muscles is complicated and often misunderstood, Chapter Four is devoted to this topic. Misconceptions and facts are presented clearly, along with a description of the anatomy and function of these muscles.

The problem of low back pain often results from poor body mechanics — the improper use of the body in positions and activities that are golf-related or work-related. Chapter Five includes suggestions about how you can use your body in ways to avoid stress and strain.

Chapter Six provides useful information specifically about the care of the back. If you have experienced back pain, you want to know how to prevent or control the problem in order to keep on playing golf. Common-sense approaches to dealing with an acute attack — and preventing a recurrence — are included in this chapter.

This book is not about how to play golf, it is about how to *stay in shape* to play golf. It is not about how to improve your golf game; it is about how to *improve your body* so you can play better, decrease the chance of injury, and keep on playing.

This book is not about how to diagnose back problems. Diagnosing back pain is a problem even for the experts. Nor is this book meant to replace seeing your doctor in the event that you injure your back. But it does aim to help you *prevent back pain*, and help you maintain or improve your ability to be fit and play better golf.

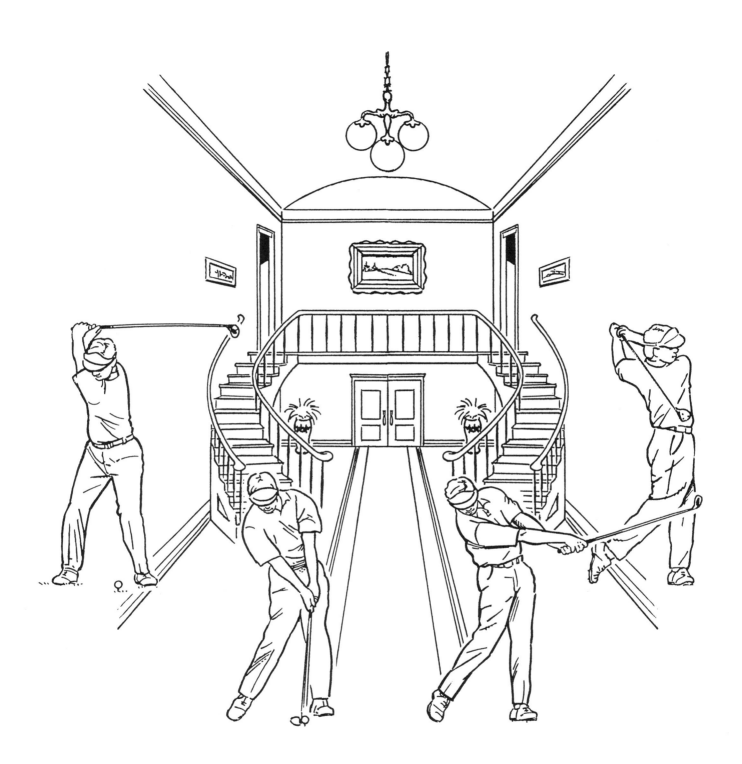

FACTS ABOUT BACKS
(Anatomy, Movements, and Positions)

For the golfer's body to meet the demands of the game, the joints of the body must allow the freedom of motion that the game requires. When movement in one or more joints is limited, there is always the danger that other joints may be strained in an effort to compensate for the lack of motion elsewhere.

Golf involves a variety of movements including forward bending, backward bending, and some side bending. But, especially, it involves rotation of the body, with the feet and head remaining in a relatively stationary position.

To help understand the rotation movements in the back-swing and the follow-through, visualize the front hall of an elegant house with two spiral staircases, one on either side, leading up to the second floor. The reason the staircase can spiral is because the shape of each step allows for some of the turning.

Now imagine that you are standing with your feet stationary and you turn your body in the direction of a spiral. There must be specific places along the way that allow for your body to turn.

Since bones do not twist, *movement must take place at various joints.*

Beginning at the feet and working up the body, you can see how the golf swing and the joint motions are related. Consider, first, the turn of the body toward the right as in the back-swing.* The right foot would naturally tend to rotate by rolling over toward the outer side, but rotation of the foot is not permitted during the back-swing because it is necessary to maintain a stable base.

Rotation does not occur in the knee joint when the knee is straight; some rotation occurs when the knee is bent. If knees are bent during the golf swing, slight rotation may occur.

The knee is not made to bend sideways. What appears to be sideways motion of the knee is really a combination of inward movement of the thigh (adduction) and rotation from the hip joint, with the knee bent.

During the golf swing, the pelvis is supposed to rotate in the same direction as the shoulders. With the feet and lower legs in fixed position, *the pelvis can only rotate as much as the hip joints will allow.*

•Throughout the book, descriptions are given for the right-handed golfer. For the left-handed golfer, simply replace the word "left" for "right" throughout the text.

MOVEMENTS OF THE SPINE

Because the pelvis is firmly attached to the spine, the spine will rotate along with the pelvis. Further rotation of the spine will allow added rotation of the shoulders, making it possible to turn the shoulders more than the pelvis.

During the golf swing, the golfer is expected to keep the head "relatively" still. The head will turn slightly toward the right during the back-swing (with eyes still on the ball), and toward the left to face the target on the follow-through. But neck rotation actually occurs as the golfer turns the shoulders in relation to the head. Neck movements must be free in order to allow the shoulders to move in relation to the fixed head position. (See below.)

Because rotation is such an important part of the golf swing, a lack of mobility can result in knee, hip, shoulder, or back problems — of which back problems appear to be the most prevalent.

In addition to rotation, forward and backward movements of the body are affected by tightness of muscles that limit joint motions and cause strain on the low back. Tight muscles in the back of the thigh (hamstrings) can interfere with forward bending by limiting the amount the hip joints will bend. Tight muscles over the front of the thigh (hip flexors) pull the low back into a forward arch (lordosis). Weakness of the abdominal muscles can also be a contributing factor in cases of low back pain. Strengthening these muscles is important in the prevention or management of low back pain. (See chapter 4.)

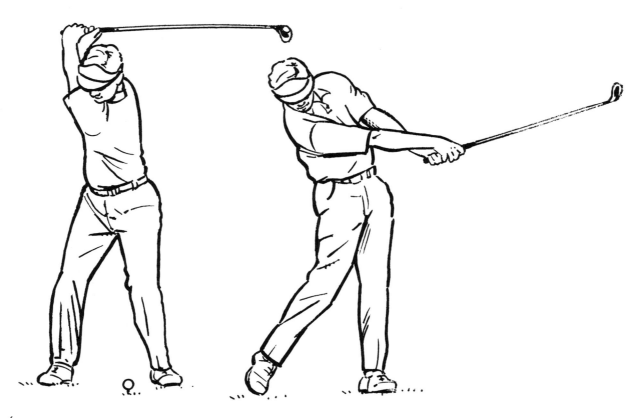

A quick anatomy lesson about the parts that make up the spinal (vertebral) column will help you understand how your back moves when you play golf.

Vertebrae are bones.

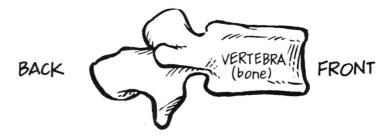

Discs are cushions that fit between the bones to allow movement and distribute pressure as the spine moves.

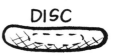

Joints exist where two bones meet and motion occurs.

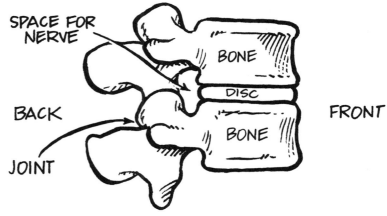

Ligaments are strong bands that hold the joints together and provide stability.

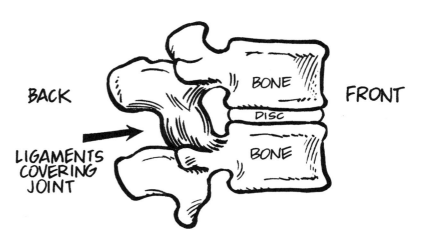

5

ANATOMY OF THE SPINE

Nerves transmit impulses to and away from the brain. They transmit messages of sensation *from* the skin and other body structures *to* the brain, and transmit messages *from* the brain *to* the muscles to make them contract.

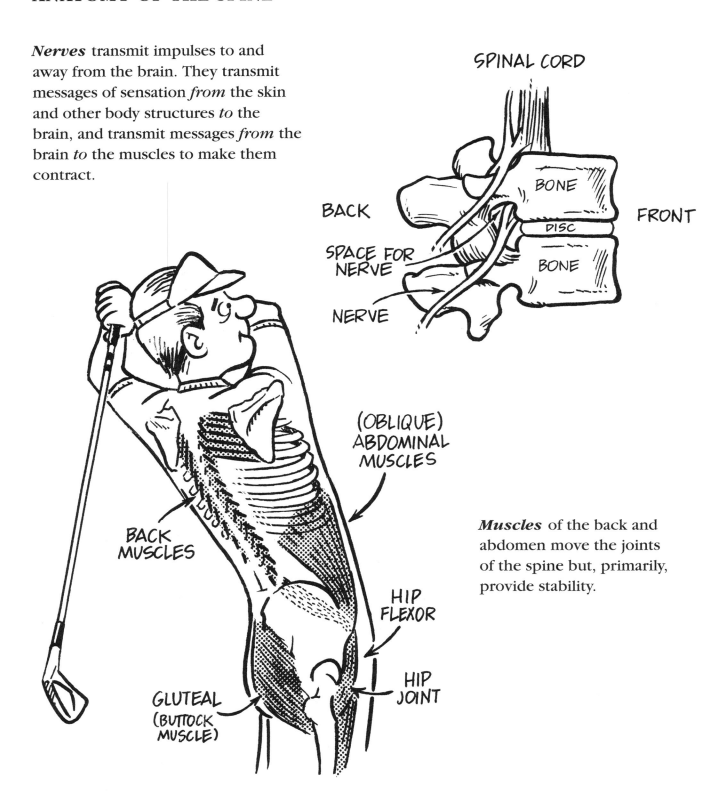

SPINAL CORD

BACK

SPACE FOR NERVE

NERVE

BONE

DISC

BONE

FRONT

(OBLIQUE) ABDOMINAL MUSCLES

BACK MUSCLES

HIP FLEXOR

HIP JOINT

GLUTEAL (BUTTOCK MUSCLE)

Muscles of the back and abdomen move the joints of the spine but, primarily, provide stability.

All these parts working together make up a complex mechanical structure that supports your body and allows you to move.

Your back is *designed* to move.

You can **bend forward** (spine flexion).

When you bend forward as far as you can, as you do when you place your tee in the ground, the front parts of the spinal column close or compress while the back parts open or stretch (A); your low back straightens and your upper back bends forward (B).

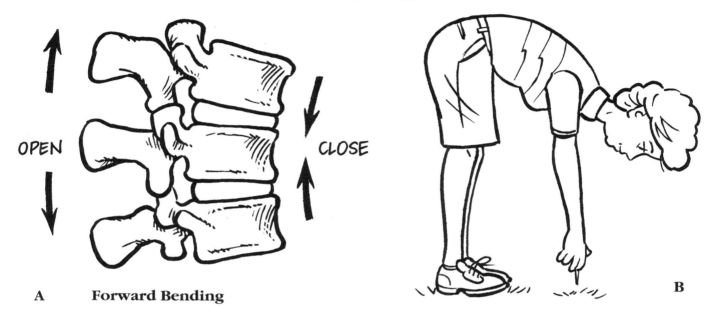

A   Forward Bending

B

You can **bend backward** (spine extension).

When you bend backward as far as you can, the back parts of your spinal column close or compress and the front parts open or stretch (C); your low back bends backward (arches) and your upper back straightens (D).

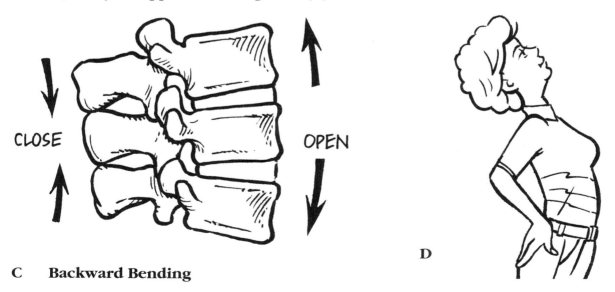

C   Backward Bending

D

MOTIONS OF THE BACK

You can **bend sideways** (lean to the side).

When you bend sideways, the side to which you bend closes or compresses and the other side opens or stretches (A). Since this motion is normally combined with rotation, greater compression and stretching occur.

You can also **rotate** (turn or twist).

When you rotate your body with your feet and legs positioned firmly, the turning motion of the pelvis and spine causes a combination of compressions and stretches.

When you combine rotation with forward bending or arching backward (as in swinging a golf club) the compressions and stretches are magnified (B).

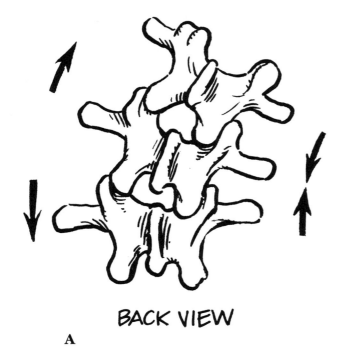

BACK VIEW

A

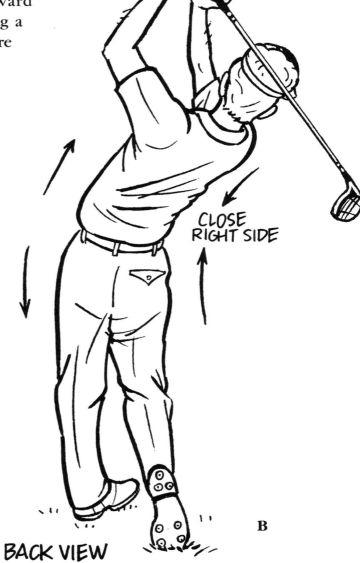

CLOSE RIGHT SIDE

BACK VIEW

B

MOTIONS OF THE BODY DURING THE GOLF SWING

The classic golf swing combines the movements of bending forward, bending backward, bending sideways, and rotating.

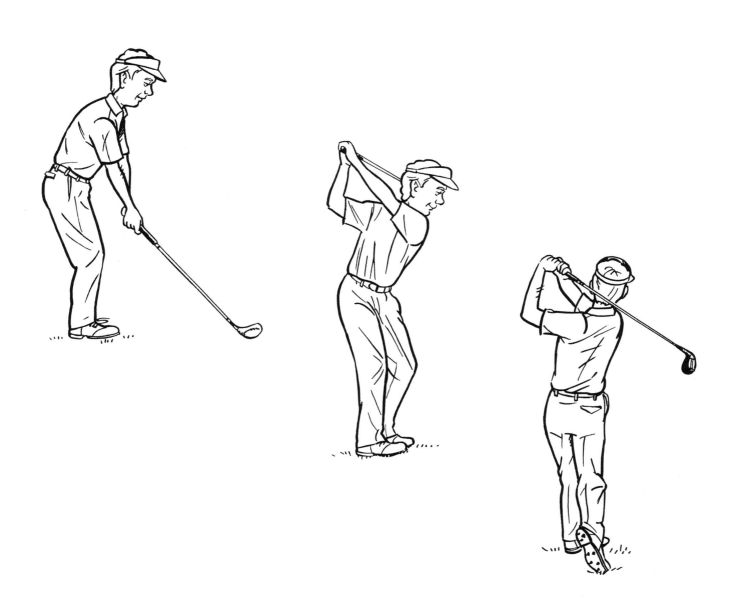

MODIFYING YOUR GOLF SWING

According to professional golfer Hale Irwin, "Physical shape and size have a direct bearing on the way a golfer builds his swing. It is important to harness what nature has given you rather than fighting against it."* Taking lessons from a golf professional can help you build your own style of swing if your physical characteristics require that you modify your game.

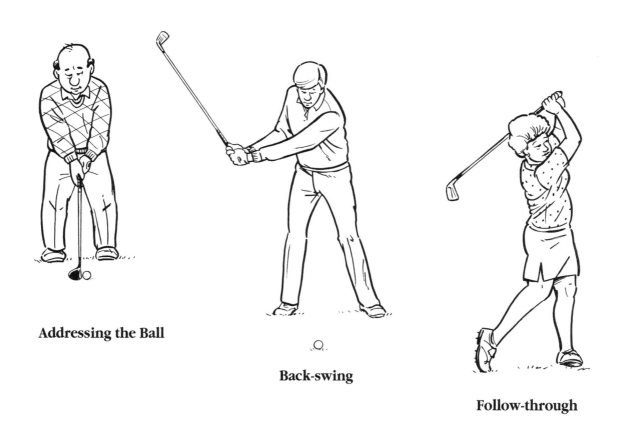

Addressing the Ball

Back-swing

Follow-through

The remainder of this chapter describes the *positions*
of various parts of the body during the classic golf swing:

1) When addressing the ball,
2) At the end of the back-swing (three views),
3) At the end of the follow-through (three views),
4) When putting.

*Hale Irwin, *Play Better Golf with Hale Irwin.* (London: Octopus Books Limited, 1980), p. 25.

Good balance in your set-up position and throughout your swing helps to protect your back. Your posture should be at ease, and be comfortable.

1) Place your hands on the club with your proper grip.

2) Position your feet apart for good balance and stability.

3) Flex your knees and hips slightly to allow rhythm and balance in your swing.

4) Incline your body slightly forward, with your low back straight.

5) Keep your upper back and neck in a neutral position.

6) Position your shoulders to allow your arms to be relaxed and "at ease." Your right shoulder will be lower than your left because your right hand is lower on your club.

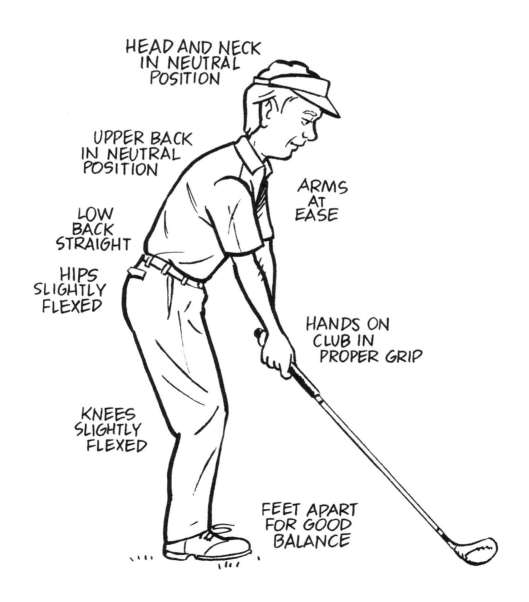

HEAD AND NECK IN NEUTRAL POSITION

UPPER BACK IN NEUTRAL POSITION

LOW BACK STRAIGHT

HIPS SLIGHTLY FLEXED

KNEES SLIGHTLY FLEXED

ARMS AT EASE

HANDS ON CLUB IN PROPER GRIP

FEET APART FOR GOOD BALANCE

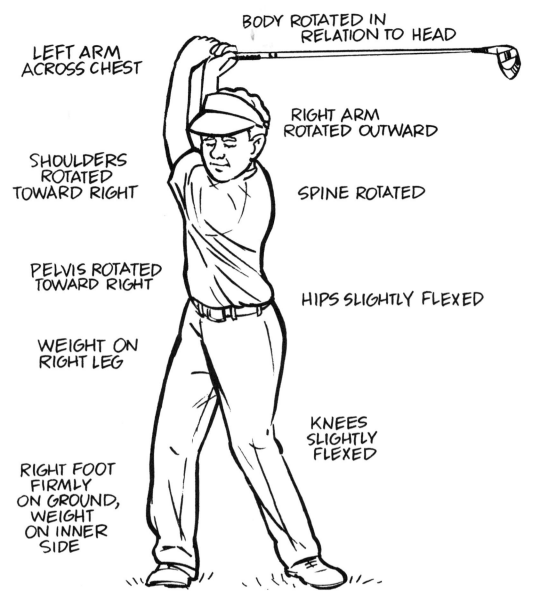

BODY ROTATED IN
RELATION TO HEAD

LEFT ARM
ACROSS CHEST

RIGHT ARM
ROTATED OUTWARD

SHOULDERS
ROTATED
TOWARD RIGHT

SPINE ROTATED

PELVIS ROTATED
TOWARD RIGHT

HIPS SLIGHTLY FLEXED

WEIGHT ON
RIGHT LEG

KNEES
SLIGHTLY
FLEXED

RIGHT FOOT
FIRMLY
ON GROUND,
WEIGHT
ON INNER
SIDE

The back-swing should be a smooth motion. To accomplish this, many parts of your body must move together.

1) Your right foot is firmly anchored to the ground so it will not rotate or slip during the coil. (The spikes on your shoes help anchor you. Without spikes your feet can slip or rotate.)

2) Your weight shifts to the right leg with your weight on the *inner side* of your right foot.

3) With your knees and hips slightly flexed, your pelvis rotates toward the right as you coil into your back-swing.

4) Your spine rotates.

5) Your right arm rotates outward.

6) Your left arm crosses your chest.

7) Your shoulders rotate toward the right. (It appears as if the head has rotated in relation to the body but, in fact, the body has rotated in relation to the head. See pp. 4 and 30.)

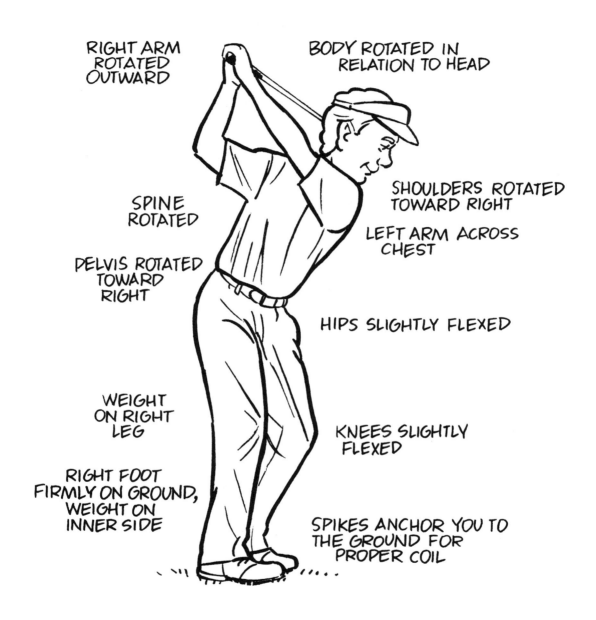

RIGHT ARM ROTATED OUTWARD

BODY ROTATED IN RELATION TO HEAD

SPINE ROTATED

SHOULDERS ROTATED TOWARD RIGHT

LEFT ARM ACROSS CHEST

PELVIS ROTATED TOWARD RIGHT

HIPS SLIGHTLY FLEXED

WEIGHT ON RIGHT LEG

KNEES SLIGHTLY FLEXED

RIGHT FOOT FIRMLY ON GROUND, WEIGHT ON INNER SIDE

SPIKES ANCHOR YOU TO THE GROUND FOR PROPER COIL

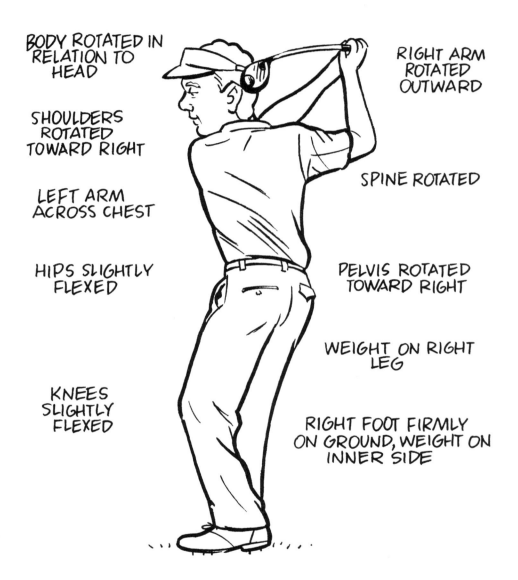

BODY ROTATED IN RELATION TO HEAD

RIGHT ARM ROTATED OUTWARD

SHOULDERS ROTATED TOWARD RIGHT

SPINE ROTATED

LEFT ARM ACROSS CHEST

HIPS SLIGHTLY FLEXED

PELVIS ROTATED TOWARD RIGHT

WEIGHT ON RIGHT LEG

KNEES SLIGHTLY FLEXED

RIGHT FOOT FIRMLY ON GROUND, WEIGHT ON INNER SIDE

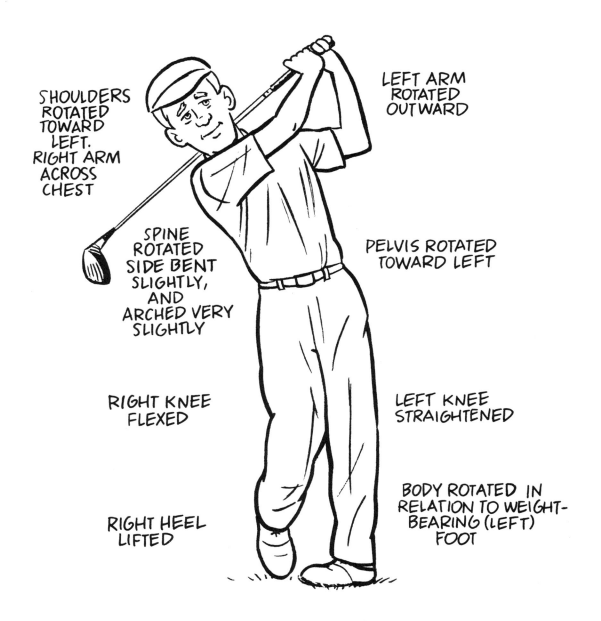

SHOULDERS ROTATED TOWARD LEFT. RIGHT ARM ACROSS CHEST

LEFT ARM ROTATED OUTWARD

SPINE ROTATED SIDE BENT SLIGHTLY, AND ARCHED VERY SLIGHTLY

PELVIS ROTATED TOWARD LEFT

RIGHT KNEE FLEXED

LEFT KNEE STRAIGHTENED

RIGHT HEEL LIFTED

BODY ROTATED IN RELATION TO WEIGHT-BEARING (LEFT) FOOT

As you follow through,

1) Your pelvis rotates toward the left.

2) Your weight shifts to the outside of your left foot and the right heel comes off the ground.

3) Your right knee flexes; your left knee straightens.

4) Your spine rotates, side-bends slightly, and arches very slightly.

5) Your left arm rotates outward.

6) Your right arm crosses your chest.

7) Your shoulders rotate toward the left. (The body has rotated in relation to the head.)

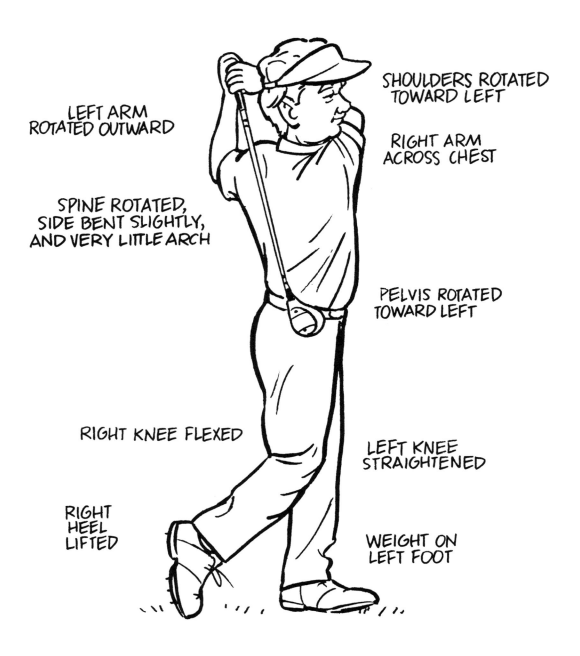

SHOULDERS ROTATED
TOWARD LEFT

LEFT ARM
ROTATED OUTWARD

RIGHT ARM
ACROSS CHEST

SPINE ROTATED,
SIDE BENT SLIGHTLY,
AND VERY LITTLE ARCH

PELVIS ROTATED
TOWARD LEFT

RIGHT KNEE FLEXED

LEFT KNEE
STRAIGHTENED

RIGHT
HEEL
LIFTED

WEIGHT ON
LEFT FOOT

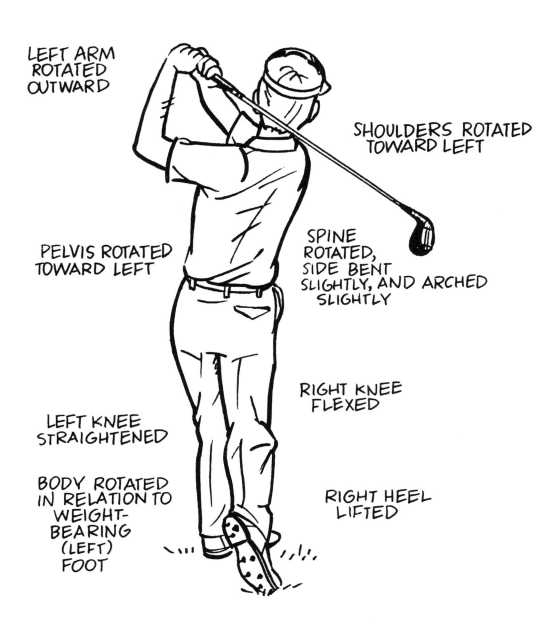

LEFT ARM ROTATED OUTWARD

SHOULDERS ROTATED TOWARD LEFT

PELVIS ROTATED TOWARD LEFT

SPINE ROTATED, SIDE BENT SLIGHTLY, AND ARCHED SLIGHTLY

RIGHT KNEE FLEXED

LEFT KNEE STRAIGHTENED

BODY ROTATED IN RELATION TO WEIGHT-BEARING (LEFT) FOOT

RIGHT HEEL LIFTED

PUTTING

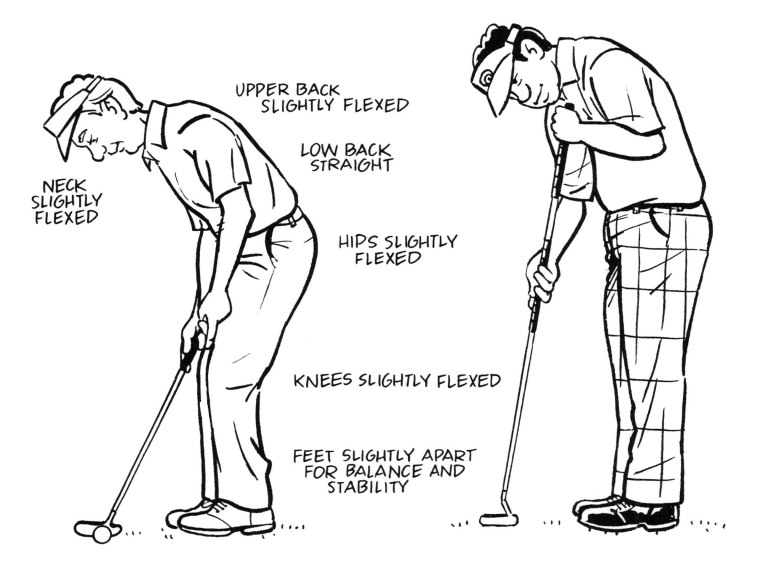

Correct putting posture is important to your game.

1) Feet are slightly apart for balance and stability.
2) Knees are slightly flexed.
3) Hips are slightly flexed.
4) Low back is straight.
5) Upper back is slightly flexed.
6) Neck is slightly flexed.

Some golfers prefer a chest-high putter. If you experience back pain when bending forward, the chest-high putter will help protect your back by limiting your forward bending.

What is your putting posture? Are your knees and hips straight or bent? Is your back too straight or too rounded?

C H A P T E R   2

WALKING AND WARM-UPS

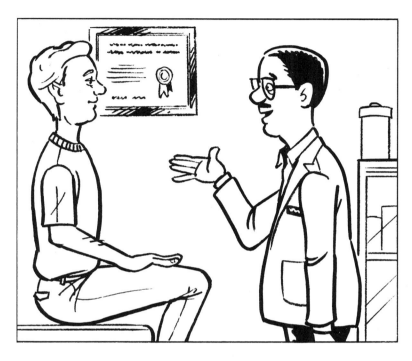

Get fit to play golf; don't play golf to get fit!

Establishing a Walking Program

You may think that you do enough walking by playing golf. However, if you use a cart, you eliminate any advantage of playing golf as a walking exercise.

Consider beginning a walking program at home on the days that you do not play golf. The strength and endurance achieved will increase your enjoyment of the game.

Walking, even at a leisurely pace, can benefit your health. Because it is a weight-bearing exercise, it helps in the prevention of osteoporosis (loss of bone density) that may occur in both men and women. A regular walking program is also good for your heart and lungs if you walk fast enough to achieve an aerobic workout. It is wise to have an annual checkup, and, for an aerobic workout, talk with your physician about your target heart rate.

CHOOSING PROPER FOOTWEAR

You should wear golf and walking shoes that are both long enough and wide enough to fit your feet. Many foot problems are due to poorly fitted shoes. If you have foot problems, see an orthopedist, podiatrist, or a physical therapist who specializes in sports medicine. You may need special inserts made for your walking shoes. The inserts should be suitable for your golf shoes also.

Ask the person who will be making your inserts whether you should wait to buy your shoes until after the inserts are made, because the shoe will need to be large enough to accommodate the insert. Be sure that the support is placed exactly where your foot needs it. You may also want to try a shock-absorbing innersole — there are many types available.

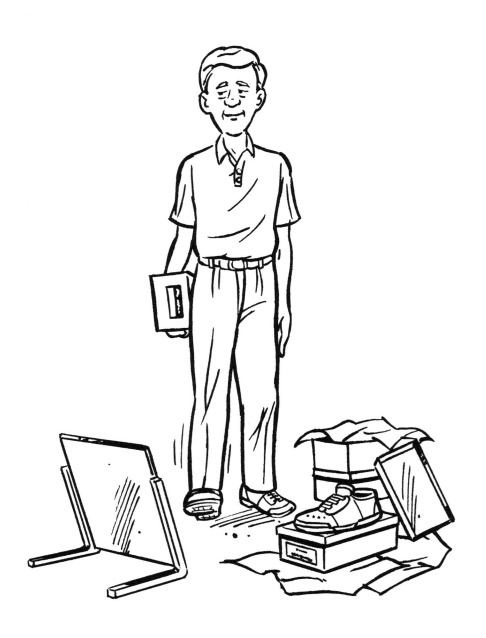

Wear shoes that have good support for your feet and have insoles that serve as cushions. Do not wear worn-out shoes. When the insoles no longer cushion as shock absorbers, the effect is felt by the legs and the spine. If the shoe is run down at the heel or broken down in the arch, postural alignment is affected.

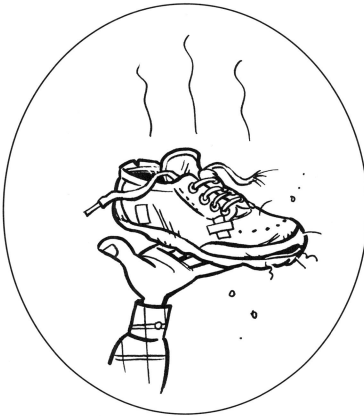

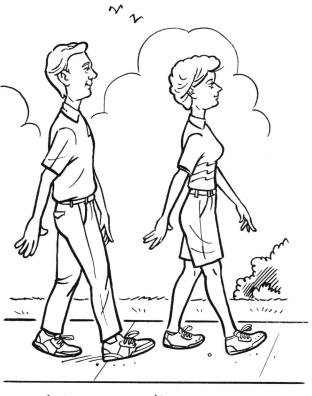

If you experience back pain when you walk, consider the following solutions:

1) Tighten your lower abdominal muscles to stabilize your spine while walking.

2) Change the length of your stride to see if you can lessen your pain.

3) Perform the flexibility exercises for your ankles, hips, and back before walking. (See exercises on pages 25, 26, and 36.)

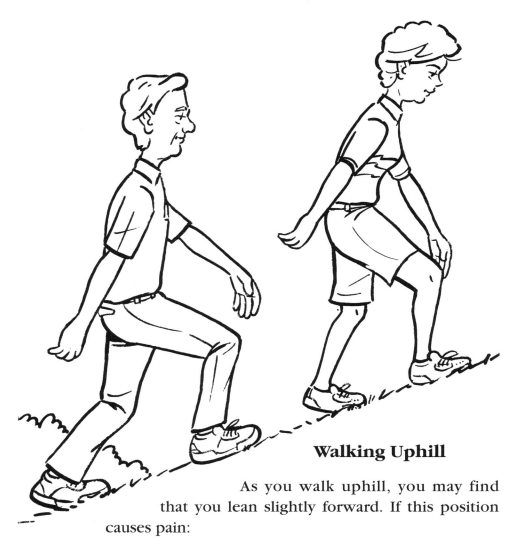

Walking Uphill

As you walk uphill, you may find that you lean slightly forward. If this position causes pain:

1) Try straightening up. Doing so will place your low back in a more natural position and will help to straighten your upper back.

2) Try changing the length of your stride. Shorter or longer steps may reduce the strain.

However, if you are holding your back too straight and your back hurts when you walk uphill, try leaning a little forward.

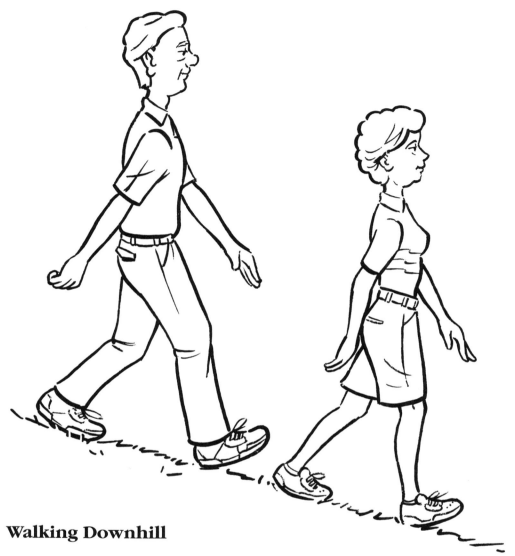

Walking Downhill

The tendency in going downhill is for your body to lean back. This increases the curve in your low back. If this position causes pain:

1) Try tightening your lower abdominal muscles. Firming these muscles provides support for your back.

2) As you step forward, avoid locking your knees. Keep a little spring in your step.

3) Try taking shorter steps and walking slower.

By walking to improve your endurance, you may also improve your golf.

WARM-UP EXERCISES

Your golf game involves movements of the spine in all directions (forward, backward, sideways, and twisting). After sitting at a desk all day or driving to the golf course, you may feel stiff and your body may not be flexible. *Do not warm up by playing a few holes.*

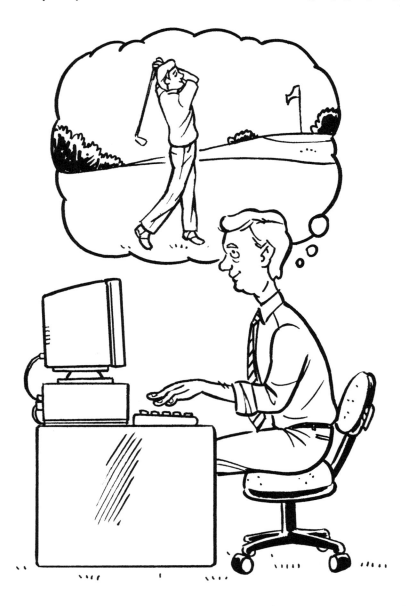

Allow time for warming up at the practice area when you arrive at the course. The following pages (25 to 30) describe eight simple warm-up exercises. The complete set can be done slowly in about eight minutes.

Do these exercises in a smooth, controlled manner (no quick, forceful, jerking movements).

1) Knee to Chest (to limber up your back and hips). Begin by standing and facing a bench. If necessary, hold on to something to help maintain your balance. Put your right foot on the seat of the bench. Lean forward, bringing your chest toward your right knee. Do this five times. Now repeat this same exercise with your left leg.

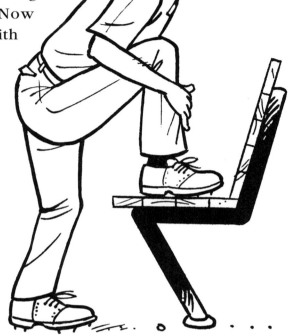

2) Modified Squat (to limber up your back, hips, and knees). Bend down in a modified squat position. Feel the stretch of your low back and hips. Repeat, reversing leg positions. Then stand up.

Do not squat if you have a problem with your knees. Instead, sit on a bench and pull one knee toward your chest. Put your leg down and pull the other knee toward your chest. Repeat five times with each leg.

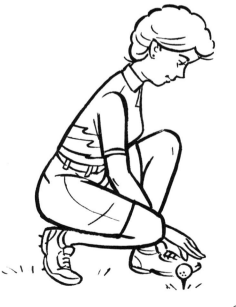

3) Back Arch (to limber up your back). This stretch into an arched position helps make your back ready for your swing. While standing, place your hands at the back of your pelvis.

Gently lean backwards, allowing your back to arch as far as comfortable and your knees to flex slightly.

Next arch your back and twist slightly to the right, then slightly to the left. If this arching motion is painful, you must limit the extent to which you arch your low back during your back-swing and follow-through.

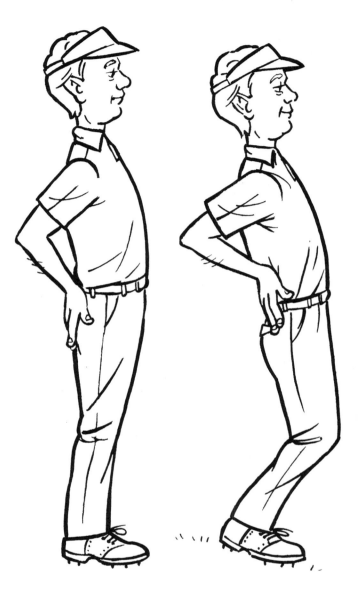

This golfer has stiffness in his back. In attempting to *bend* backward he can only *lean* backward by bending at the knees and ankles. Doing the exercise this way will not improve the flexibility of his back.

4) Shoulder Stretch (to limber up your shoulders). Stand with your feet comfortably apart, knees "at ease," with your lower abdominal muscles firm to hold your spine stable. Hold your club horizontally:

a) Raise your arms up overhead five to ten times. Do not arch your low back to bring the club higher. (See page 58.)

b) Raise your arms to shoulder height and move your arms across your chest to the right and to the left, five times each way. (Do not turn your body — only stretch your shoulders.)

c) Repeat the above exercise — only this time, when moving arms to the right, gently turn your head to the left; when moving your arms to the left, gently turn your head to the right. Do the exercise five times each way.

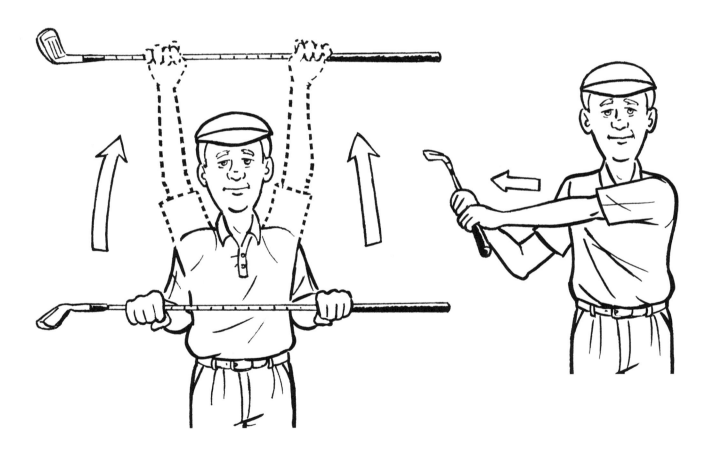

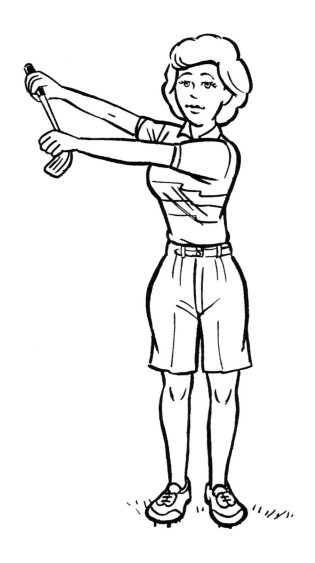

5) Rotation (to limber up your spine). This twisting motion helps you prepare for a full swing. Begin with your feet comfortably apart and firmly planted on the ground. Your knees should be in neutral position (eased) and kneecaps should face directly forward. Make your lower abdominal muscles firm. Hold your club horizontally in both hands, and bring it to shoulder level. Slowly rotate your upper body toward the *right* (to limber up your back for your back-swing). Now slowly rotate to your *left* (to limber up your back for your follow-through).

Repeat the exercise five times each way.

6) Full Rotation

Combine exercises #4 and #5 with rotation of the hips for full flexibility of your hips, back, and arms.

1) Rotate your pelvis to the right; turn your shoulders to the right, and stretch your arms to the right.

2) Hold for five seconds.

3) Reverse the motion, rotating your pelvis to the left, turning your shoulders to the left, and stretching your arms to the left.

4) Hold for five seconds.

5) Repeat the exercise five times to each side.

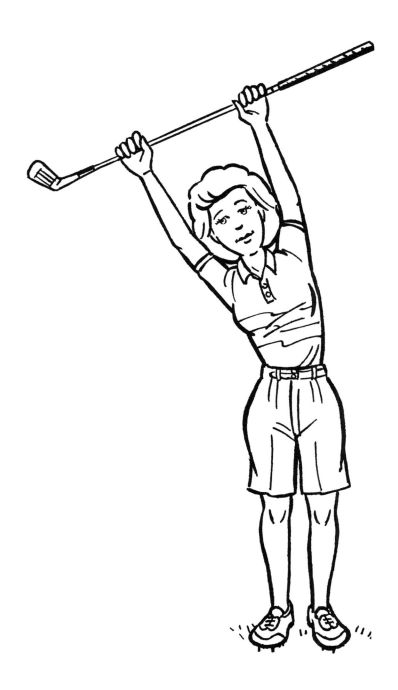

7) Side Bends (to limber up your spine in a side-bending motion).

Stand with your feet comfortably apart, knees unlocked, and your lower abdominal muscles firm. Hold your club overhead and bend from side to side. Do five stretches to each side.

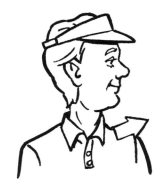 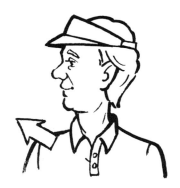 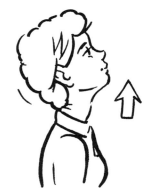

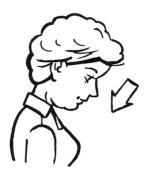

8) Neck Motions (to limber up your neck).

Stand with your feet comfortably apart, knees at ease, lower abdominal muscles firm, and upper back straight. *Keep your shoulders facing forward* and turn your head, first to the left, and then to the right, as far as comfortable. Repeat this exercise five times to each side.

With your shoulders facing forward, move your head to look up and look down. Repeat this exercise five times.

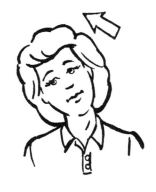

Now move your head sideways to bring your left ear toward your left shoulder. Then move your head to bring your right ear toward your right shoulder. Repeat each exercise five times.

Remember, in golf you are instructed to keep your eyes on the ball. In order to keep facing forward with your eyes on the ball as your shoulders turn *right into your back-swing,* you must have a good range of rotation motion in your *neck.* The amount of neck rotation required is the same as the amount of rotation needed to turn your head to look over your left shoulder when your shoulders are facing forward.

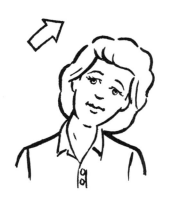

SELF-TESTS AND EXERCISES

In order to play golf and feel your best, you need the flexibility and strength required for your golf swing.

This chapter includes self-tests that can help you determine if you lack flexibility or strength. The results of the self-tests will help you decide what exercises are most appropriate for you.

The following three illustrations point out some of the specific motions of joints and strength of muscles that you need to complete your swing.

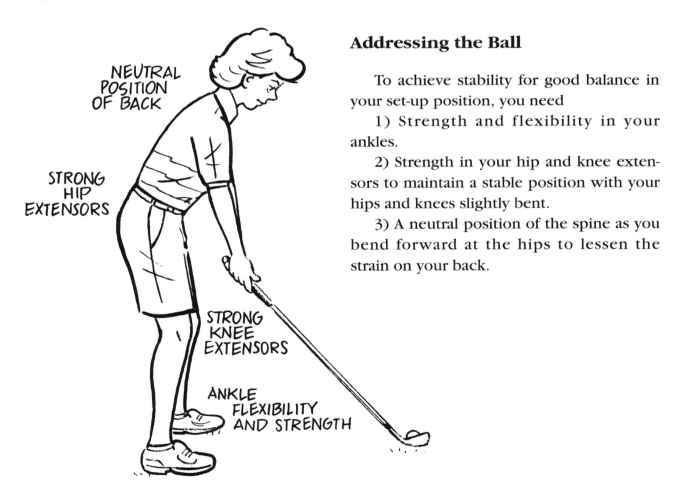

NEUTRAL
POSITION
OF BACK

STRONG
HIP
EXTENSORS

STRONG
KNEE
EXTENSORS

ANKLE
FLEXIBILITY
AND STRENGTH

Addressing the Ball

To achieve stability for good balance in your set-up position, you need

1) Strength and flexibility in your ankles.

2) Strength in your hip and knee extensors to maintain a stable position with your hips and knees slightly bent.

3) A neutral position of the spine as you bend forward at the hips to lessen the strain on your back.

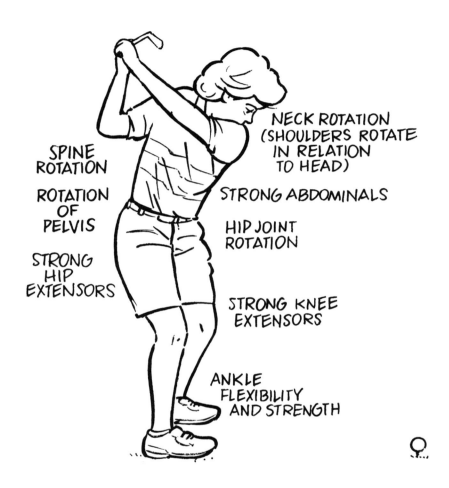

SPINE
ROTATION

ROTATION
OF
PELVIS

STRONG
HIP
EXTENSORS

NECK ROTATION
(SHOULDERS ROTATE
IN RELATION
TO HEAD)

STRONG ABDOMINALS

HIP JOINT
ROTATION

STRONG KNEE
EXTENSORS

ANKLE
FLEXIBILITY
AND STRENGTH

For your back-swing, you need

1) Strength in your ankles for stability; strength and flexibility in your ankles in order to shift your body weight.

2) Strength in your hip and knee extensors to support you in the knee-bent position.

3) Flexibility in your hip joints, especially in rotation. As the pelvis rotates toward the right, the right hip joint rotates inward and the left hip joint rotates outward. (See p. 50.)

4) Strength in your abdominal muscles to provide support for your trunk.

5) Strength in the muscles that extend and rotate your trunk and neck.

6) Flexibility and strength in your shoulders in order to bring your club to the top of your back-swing.

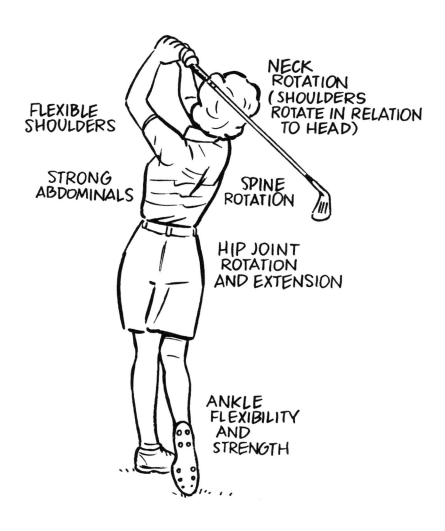

NECK ROTATION (SHOULDERS ROTATE IN RELATION TO HEAD)

FLEXIBLE SHOULDERS

STRONG ABDOMINALS

SPINE ROTATION

HIP JOINT ROTATION AND EXTENSION

ANKLE FLEXIBILITY AND STRENGTH

For your follow-through, you need

1) Strength and flexibility in your ankles.

2) Flexibility of your hips in extension to allow you to straighten your hips without pulling your spine into an excessive arch.

3) Flexibility in hip rotation — inward rotation of the left hip joint and outward rotation of the right hip joint. (See p. 50.)

4) Flexibility of your spine in back-bending, rotation, and side-bending.

5) Strength in your back and abdominal muscles to maintain stabilization of your trunk and help prevent excessive motion of your spine.

6) Flexibility of your neck and shoulders.

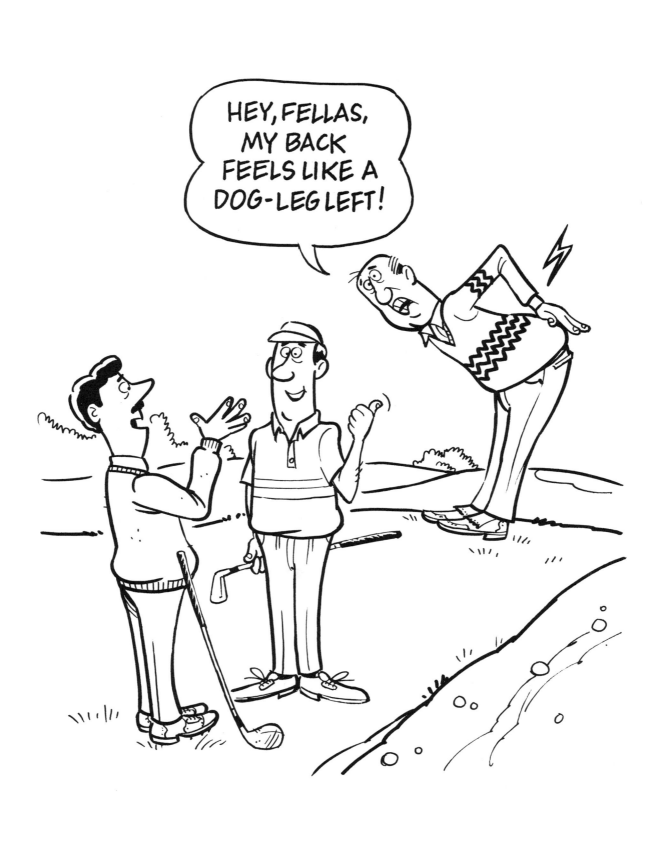

Joint or muscle tightness in your ankles, hips, shoulders, neck, or back will limit your ability to rotate into your backswing or follow-through. Do not try to compensate for tightness in one area by overstretching another area.

If your body feels stiff and your muscles are tight, you need exercises for flexibility. Some of the tightness may be in the joints as well as in the muscles. If a joint does not have any arthritic changes, the chances are that it will loosen up as the muscles stretch. If your muscles are weak, you need exercises to improve your strength and stability. Do the tests and the exercises slowly and carefully. *You may feel some mild discomfort, but you should not feel pain when doing either the tests or the exercises. If they cause pain, stop doing them.*

You do not need to perform all of these tests in one day. Try two or three at a time. If you do not feel able to do these self-tests you may want to seek help from a physical therapist who has expertise in musculo-skeletal testing.

It is possible that muscles may become weak by over-stretching as well as inflexible by over-strengthening. When you are stretching muscles, do the exercises in a slow, controlled manner to help protect you from over-stretching or tearing muscle fibers. Such injury can be very painful and keep you from playing golf.

Think in terms of improving your flexibility "a degree a day," and remember that some exercises are done to *maintain* your flexibility rather than to increase it.

The exercises should be done on a padded floor, about four times a week. Begin with three to five repetitions of each exercise and progress to ten. The number of repetitions may seem low, but golfers are highly motivated and often over-do.

Try to breathe normally as you exercise; do not hold your breath.

Do not wear tight clothing when you exercise because it will restrict your motion. The same advice holds true when playing golf: tight slacks limit the bend of your hips and a tight blouse or shirt limits the motion of your shoulders.

There may be tightness in joint structures that does not improve by trying to stretch the muscles. You may need to accommodate for your weakness, tightness, or lack of joint motion. In such cases, maximize your power by working within your body limits so that you will maintain control of your swing and lessen the chances of hurting yourself.

LENGTH OF CALF MUSCLES

Calf muscles are located at the back of the lower leg. The gastrocnemius muscle crosses over the ankle joint and knee joint; the soleus crosses over the ankle joint only. Do these tests with your shoes off.

Self-Test for Length of Gastrocnemius Muscle

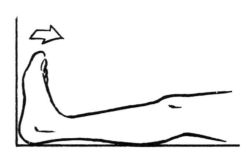

With your knee straight, pull your left foot up as far as possible. You should be able to move your foot about 10° past the right angle. Repeat self-test with your right foot.

Exercise to Stretch Tight Gastrocnemius Muscle

Stand facing a wall, at arms' length away, with your left foot forward and your right foot back as illustrated below. Allow your feet to toe out slightly. Keeping your right hip and knee straight, lean toward the wall until you feel a stretch in the right calf muscles. Hold for ten seconds and relax; repeat five times. Reverse leg positions to stretch the left calf muscles.

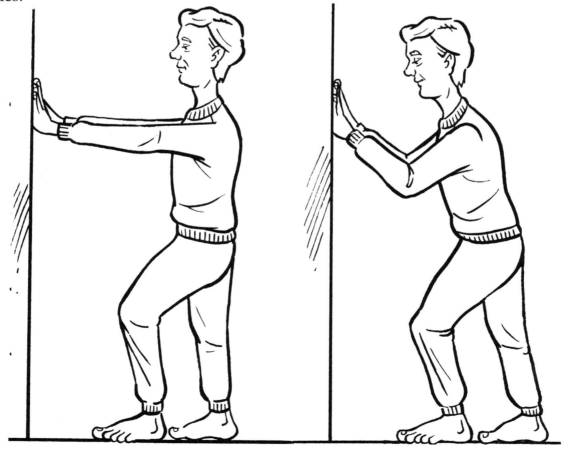

Self-Test for Length of Soleus Muscle

Sit forward on a chair or stool. Be sure the height allows your bare feet to rest comfortably on the floor. Allow your feet to toe out slightly. Keeping your heels in contact with the floor, slide your left foot back. You should be able to bend your ankle about twenty degrees past a right angle, as illustrated below. If you can keep your heel on the floor and bring the foot back so that your toes are in line with the front of your knee, you probably have about 20° of bend at the ankle.

Exercise to Stretch Tight Soleus Muscle

Use the position illustrated below. Slide both feet back until your heels come up slightly from the floor. With your hands, press down on both thighs to help push your heels down to the floor. Hold ten seconds, then relax. Repeat five times. You may do the exercise several times a day; try it at your desk if your chair is the right height.

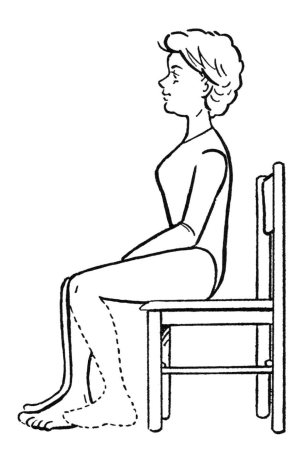

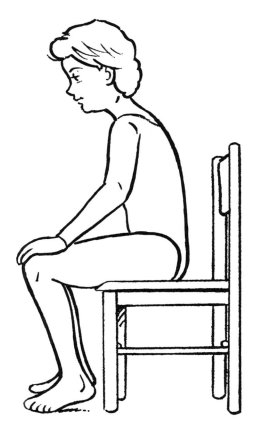

TIGHT CALF MUSCLES: EFFECT ON GOLFERS

Tightness of the calf muscles may affect your walking by restricting normal ankle motion. Women who consistently wear high heels may develop tight calf muscles.

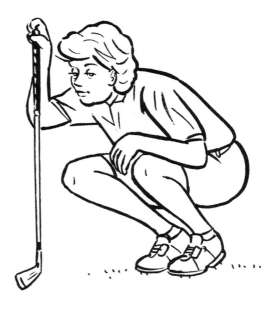

If your calf muscles are tight, you will not have the flexibility you need to keep your heels on the ground when you bend your knees to address the golf ball correctly.

If the muscles are resistant to stretch, it is possible to accomodate for the tightness by putting a lift on the heel of your shoe, or by placing a heel cushion (probably about three-sixteenths of an inch thick) inside the shoe.

For the golfer, this adjustment permits more knee bend while allowing the shoe to remain in contact with the ground. Permitting this stance is particularly important while addressing the ball or putting.

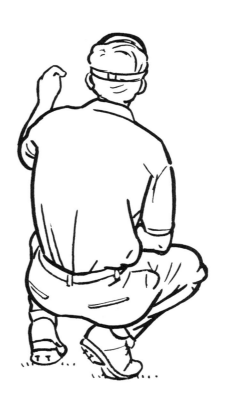

To squat, your ankles as well as your hips and knees must be able to bend freely. If the ankles do not bend as much as they should, more bend will take place at the fore-foot, resulting in stretch, strain, and pressure on the front of the foot.

The following page shows exercises to increase flexibility of the hips and knees.

Self-Test for Hip and Knee Flexion

Most people have good flexibility in bending hips and knees. To test for your range of motion, do the following.

Starting Position: Lie on your back with your knees bent and your feet resting on the floor. Use a pillow under your head if needed for comfort.

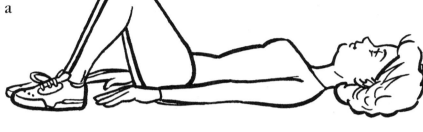

Try to bring your left knee to your chest with the knee bent. If you cannot do this as illustrated, you probably have limited motion.

Exercise for Hip and Knee Flexion

If your motion is limited, use the following exercise to increase your range of motion. Bring your left knee toward your chest, gently pull with your arms, and hold for five seconds. Return your left leg to the starting position and repeat with your right leg. Repeat five times with each leg.

Next, bring both knees to your chest and hold for a count of ten seconds. Return left leg to the starting position; then return your right leg to starting position and repeat five times.

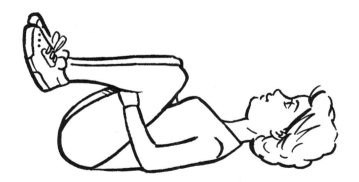

Effect on Golfers

If your hip and knee flexion are limited, you will have difficulty doing such things as squatting and tying your shoes.

HIP AND KNEE EXTENSORS

Hip extensors (gluteals) are located on the back of the hip; and knee extensors (quadriceps) are located on the front of the thigh.

Self-Test for Strength of Hip and Knee Extensors

If you know that you are able to squat and get up easily (without using your hands to push or pull yourself up), you have good strength in your hip and knee extensors; if you know that you cannot do this, do *not* attempt to do these motions as a test.

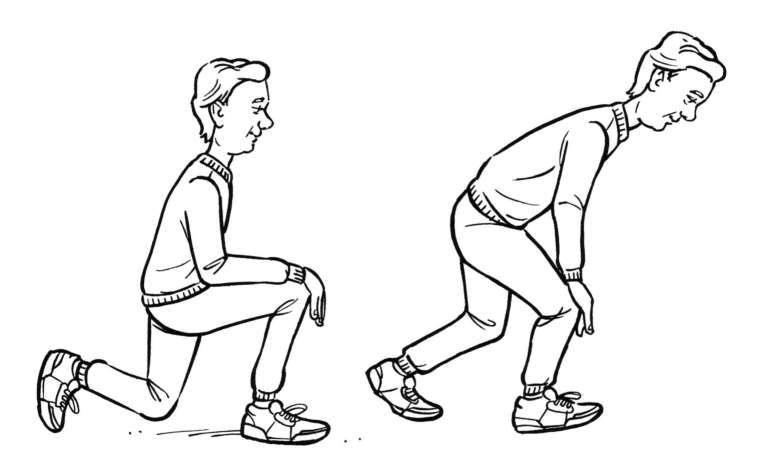

If you need "self-assistance" by pushing with your hand (as illustrated above) or holding on to something to pull yourself up, you can be helped by the simple exercise described on p. 41.

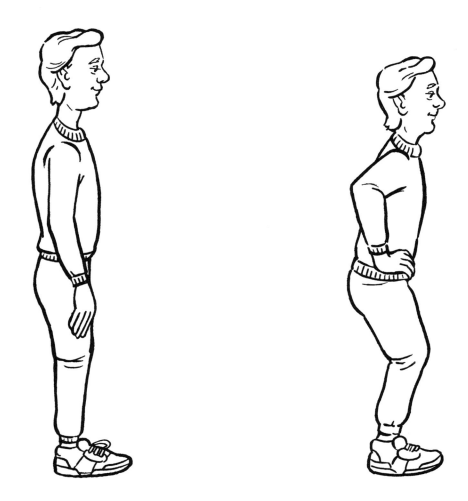

Exercise to Strengthen Hip and Knee Extensors

Start by standing up straight. Bend your hips and knees slightly, inclining your upper body slightly forward as illustrated. Hold for five seconds. Stand up, and repeat ten times. This exercise begins with the slight knee-bend and works up to a moderate bend. Do not go into a deep knee-bend (past a ninety-degree bend of the knee).

Stair climbing is also a good exercise for hip and knee extensors.

Effect on Golfers

As a golfer, you need strong hip and knee extensors in order to hold the hips and knees slightly bent when addressing the ball and putting.

To raise your body up from a squat position you need very strong hip and knee extensors. In addition there are many ordinary activities associated with golf that require bending and straightening the hips and knees, such as picking up your bag, placing the ball on the tee, lining up your putt, and picking up the ball from the cup.

LENGTH OF HIP FLEXORS

The hip flexor muscles cross the front of the hip joint. They actually extend from the spine in the area of the low back and the pelvis across the front of the hip joint to the bone of the thigh (femur).

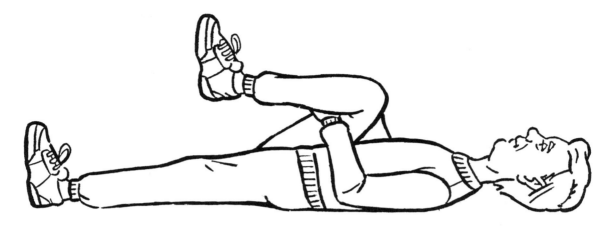

Self-Test for Length of Hip Flexors

Lie on your back with both legs straight. Bring your right knee toward your chest in order to flatten the low back. Hold firmly as illustrated above. Press the left thigh downward toward the floor. If your thigh does not touch the floor, you probably have some tightness in the left hip flexors as illustrated below. Repeat this self-test with the right leg.

Exercise to Stretch Tight Hip Flexors

Use the test as an exercise to stretch the tight hip flexors. Bring your right knee to your chest in order to flatten your back.

Extend your left leg as straight as possible. Tighten your buttock muscle and firmly press your thigh down toward the floor trying to straighten your left hip and knee. (See below. *Be sure to keep your low back flat.* Hold for a count of ten seconds. Relax and repeat with the right leg. Return to starting position and repeat with each leg five times.

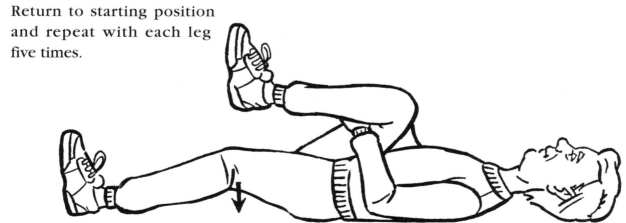

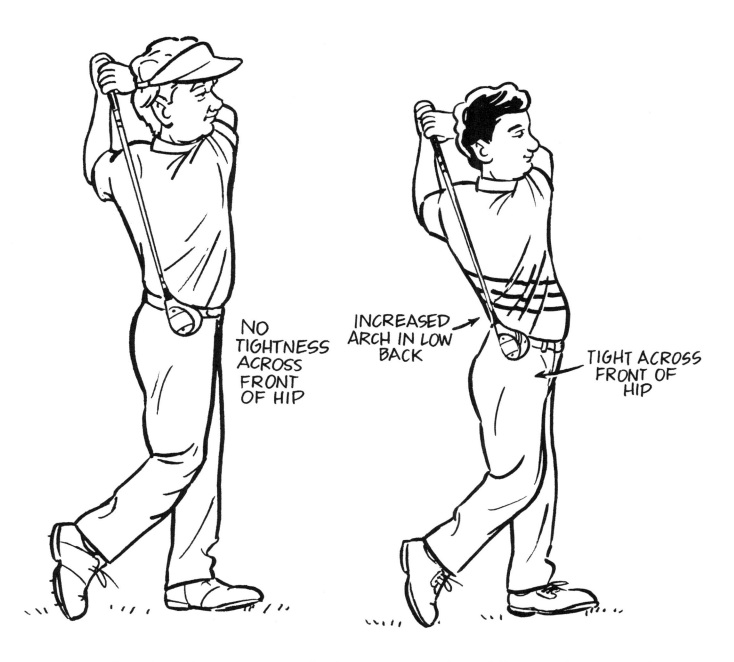

NO TIGHTNESS ACROSS FRONT OF HIP

INCREASED ARCH IN LOW BACK

TIGHT ACROSS FRONT OF HIP

The follow-through requires that the hip joints straighten fully. In order to straighten, the muscles over the front of the hip joint (hip flexors) must not be tight.

Both your standing posture and your golf swing may be significantly affected if the hip flexors are tight. Because the hip flexors attach to both the pelvis and the low back, tightness of the hip flexors can cause your low back to arch as you straighten your hips during follow-through. Extreme arching of the low back can cause serious back problems. If your hip flexors are tight, avoid injury by limiting the extent of your follow-through.

LENGTH OF HAMSTRINGS

Hamstring muscles are located at the back of the thigh, crossing the hip joint and the knee joint.

Self-Test for Length of Hamstrings

Lie on your back with legs out straight. *Keep your low back flat on the floor* and raise your left leg upward, keeping the knee straight. Let the foot relax. If you are not able to get your back flat with the legs out straight, let the right hip and knee bend *just enough* to get the back flat.

You should be able to raise your leg up almost to a vertical position. If you cannot raise your leg up to about an eighty degree angle from the floor, you probably have tight hamstrings.

Repeat the self-test with the right leg.

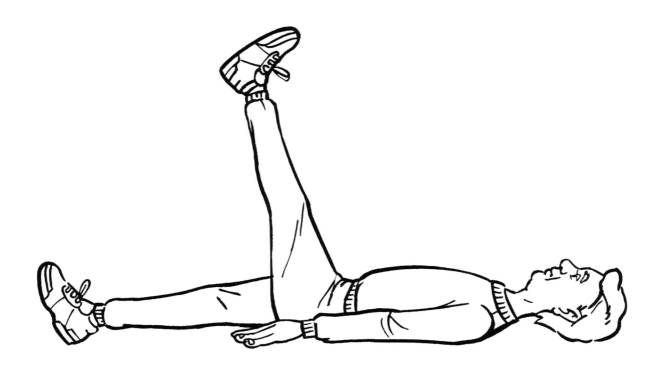

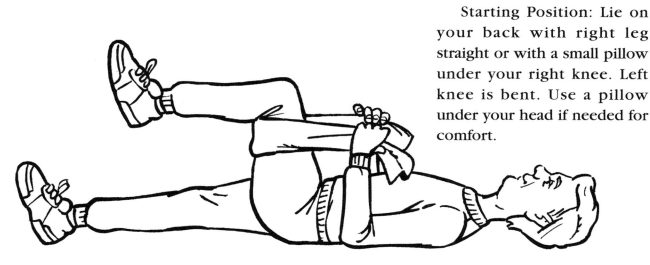

Exercise to Stretch Tight Hamstrings

Starting Position: Lie on your back with right leg straight or with a small pillow under your right knee. Left knee is bent. Use a pillow under your head if needed for comfort.

1) Place a folded towel around your left thigh like a sling, holding the ends of the towel with your hands. Brace your elbows at your sides. Support your thigh at about an eighty degree angle.

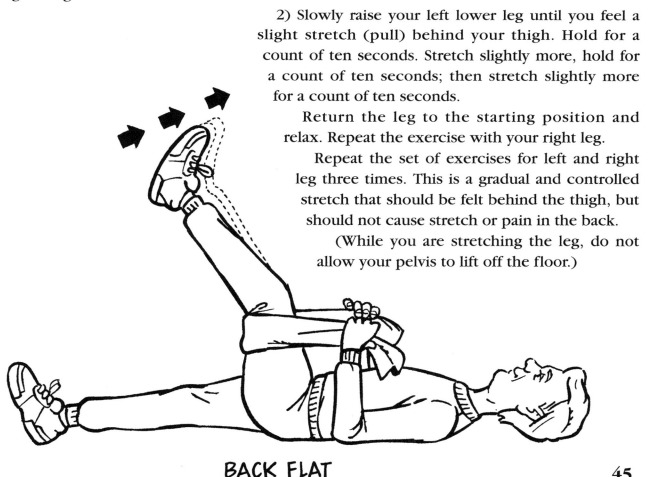

2) Slowly raise your left lower leg until you feel a slight stretch (pull) behind your thigh. Hold for a count of ten seconds. Stretch slightly more, hold for a count of ten seconds; then stretch slightly more for a count of ten seconds.

Return the leg to the starting position and relax. Repeat the exercise with your right leg.

Repeat the set of exercises for left and right leg three times. This is a gradual and controlled stretch that should be felt behind the thigh, but should not cause stretch or pain in the back.

(While you are stretching the leg, do not allow your pelvis to lift off the floor.)

BACK FLAT

HAMSTRING STRETCH IN LYING AND SITTING POSITIONS

Hamstring Stretch in Lying Position

Lie on the floor at an open doorway with your left leg out straight. Raise your right leg and rest it against the door frame at a height that gives a slight stretch behind your thigh. Hold for thirty seconds. As your muscles relax, you can inch your hips closer to the doorway to raise the leg higher and get more stretch. Hold for thirty seconds. Repeat with the other leg.

Hamstring Stretch in Sitting Position

Sit up straight and concentrate on holding your spine straight. (Do not let your back arch or slouch.)

Gradually straighten your left knee until you feel a stretch (pull) behind your thigh. Hold this position for ten seconds; relax. Alternate right and left legs, repeating the exercise five times for each leg. This is a good exercise to do anytime you are sitting in a chair.

When you bend forward from a standing position, both the hip joints and the back bend. Hamstring muscle tightness will not allow you to bend fully at the hip joints. You will have difficulty reaching toward your feet as in picking up your ball. Straining to do so will put stress on the back and may cause rounding of the low back.

If your hamstrings are not tight, you will be able to bend at your hips and not overstretch and strain your low back when you bend forward.

If you have been unable to stretch your hamstrings, you can accommodate for this tightness by bending as shown below.

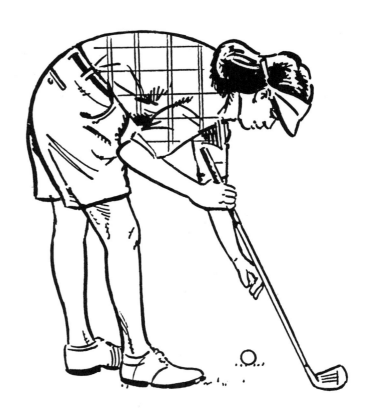

Bending with Tight Hamstrings

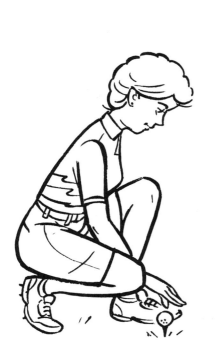

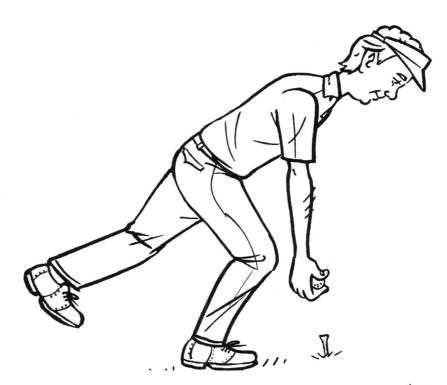

HIP JOINT ROTATION IN SITTING

Self-Test for Hip Joint Rotation, Sitting

Sit on a bench or chair that is deep enough from front to back to support the thighs.

As you do these tests, look at your legs to decide what amount of motion you have in your hips by comparing yourself to the illustration. It is not unusual to have one of your hips more flexible than the other. If you cannot rotate your hips as shown below, you probably are tight and should exercise. Do not strain to hold the test position.

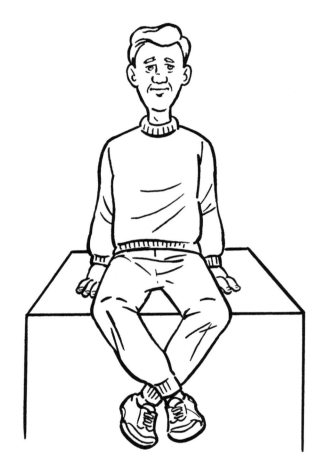 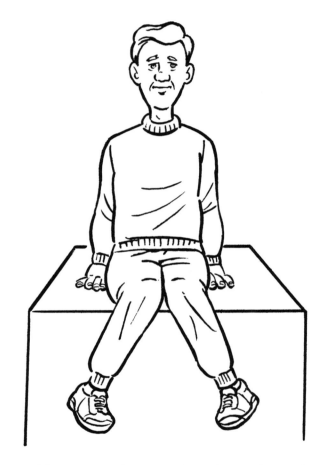

Self-Test and Exercise for Hip Joint Outward Rotation

Roll your thighs outward and cross your legs above the ankles. If your thighs cannot turn out as shown above, you should try to improve your outward rotation by exercising in this test position. Turn your thighs outward. Hold for five seconds. Relax and repeat five times.

Self-Test and Exercise for Hip Joint Inward Rotation

Keep your knees together, roll your thighs inward, and separate your feet as much as you can. If your thighs cannot turn inward as shown above, you should try to improve your inward rotation by exercising in this test position. Turn your thighs inward. Hold for five seconds. Relax and repeat five times.

Note: When doing the following test and exercise, be sure that the *thighs* are turning inward and outward. It is possible to fool yourself by turning your foot inward at the ankle joint so it appears that your leg has rolled inward more than it actually has. Check your motion by looking at your knees to see, by the position of your kneecaps, whether your thighs turn inward or outward.

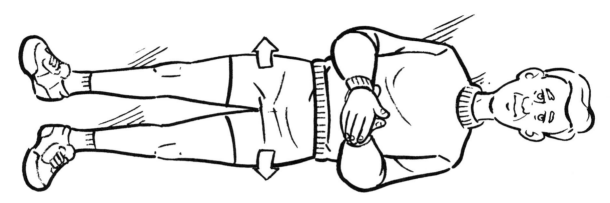

Self-Test and Exercise for Hip Joint Outward Rotation

Starting Position: Lie on your back with both legs straight. Use a pillow under your head if you need it for comfort.

Roll both legs outward to determine if you have good motion in outward rotation. Your knee-caps should face outward as illustrated above. If you are limited in this motion, use the test as an exercise. Roll legs outward and hold for five seconds. Relax and repeat five times.

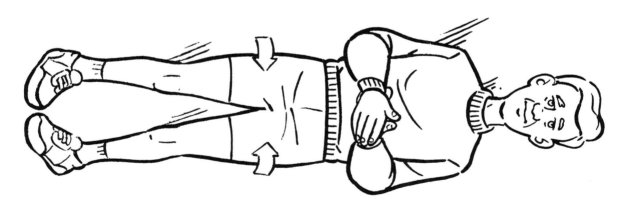

Self-Test and Exercise for Hip Joint Inward Rotation

Roll both legs inward to determine if you have good motion in inward rotation. Your knee-caps should face inward as in this illustration. If you are limited in this motion, use the test as an exercise. Roll legs inward and hold for five seconds. Relax and repeat five times.

Combine both of these motions: Roll legs inward and hold for five seconds. Roll legs outward and hold for five seconds. Repeat five times in both directions.

HIP JOINT ROTATION: EFFECT ON GOLFERS

The hip joint connects the thigh bone (femur) to the pelvis. The joint allows movement forward (flexion), backward (extension), sideways (abduction and adduction), and rotation (inward and outward). All the movements except rotation have been described elsewhere.

Understanding rotation of the hip joints in relation to the golf swing is a very important concept that is not easily described in non-technical terms. The difficulty arises because, instead of being able to describe which way the thigh rotates in relation to a fixed pelvis, the rotation of the golf swing must be described on the basis of how the pelvis rotates in relation to fixed leg positions.

Back-swing

The feet and legs are in a (relatively) stationary position.

The pelvis turns toward the right.

This results in *inward rotation* of the *right* hip joint and *outward rotation* of the *left* hip joint. (See p. 51A.)

During the back-swing, there will be less outward rotation of the left hip joint if the left heel is lifted than if it is kept on the ground.

If you have limited outward rotation of the left hip joint, you can accommodate for that limitation by allowing the left heel to come up during the back-swing because this allows the whole body to turn slightly.

Follow-through

The left foot is in a (relatively) stationary position.

The pelvis turns toward the left to face the target.

This results in *inward rotation* of the *left* hip joint and *outward* rotation of the *right* hip joint. (Less outward rotation of the right hip will occur at the end of the follow-through because as the right heel lifts off the ground the right leg is free to turn with the pelvis; see p. 51B.)

If your hip joint motion is limited and cannot be improved by exercise, it is still advisable to do the exercise to help maintain whatever range of motion you have. You will probably be better off to limit the range of your golf swing so that you will maintain control and consistency of your swing.

It is not uncommon to find that some individuals have more range of motion in outward rotation than in inward. Sometimes there is more than average motion in outward rotation and less than average in inward rotation, but the full range of motion may be as much as one who has average range in both directions.

If you, as a golfer, are limited in inward rotation of the right hip joint but you have more than average outward rotation, you will find that when you address the ball with your feet directly forward, your back-swing will be limited. (Remember, the right hip joint inwardly rotates for the back-swing.) However, if your right leg is set toeing out slightly at address position, this will allow a slight increase in your back-swing. This increase in range may be enough to make a difference in your ability to accelerate into your down-swing. However, do not sacrifice control for the ability to increase your back-swing.

HIP JOINT ROTATION IN BACK-SWING AND FOLLOW-THROUGH

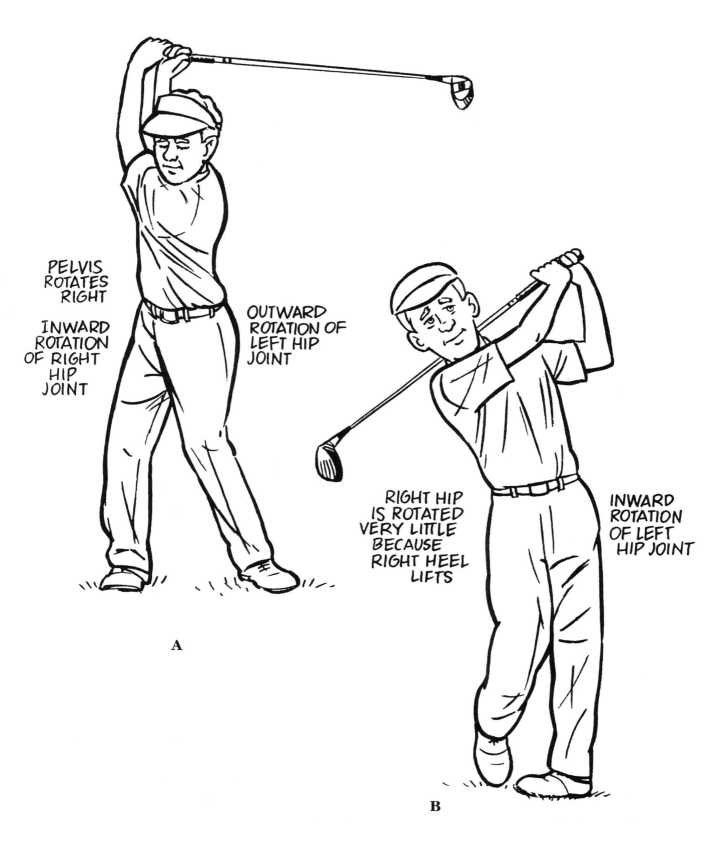

PELVIS
ROTATES
RIGHT

INWARD
ROTATION
OF RIGHT
HIP
JOINT

OUTWARD
ROTATION OF
LEFT HIP
JOINT

RIGHT HIP
IS ROTATED
VERY LITTLE
BECAUSE
RIGHT HEEL
LIFTS

INWARD
ROTATION
OF LEFT
HIP JOINT

A

B

SPINE ROTATION

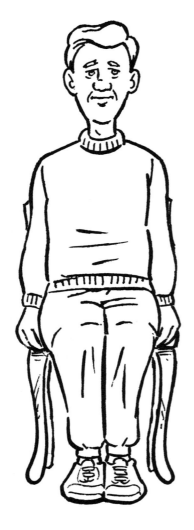
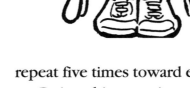

Self-Test and Exercise for Spine Rotation

To rotate the spine without rotating the pelvis, do the following. Sit on a bench or chair deep enough from front to back to completely support the thighs. Keep your knees bent over the edge of the seat. Sitting with your back straight, arms down at your sides, turn your body slowly toward the right as far as comfortable. (Do not strain to turn.) Then repeat slowly toward the left. Hold each turn for about five seconds, and repeat five times toward each side.

Doing this exercise will help you maintain or increase your spine rotation for your golf swing and strengthen your oblique abdominal muscles.

Effect on Golfers

The amount of rotation of the spine varies a good deal from one person to another. For golfers, spine rotation is especially important for your back-swing and follow-through.

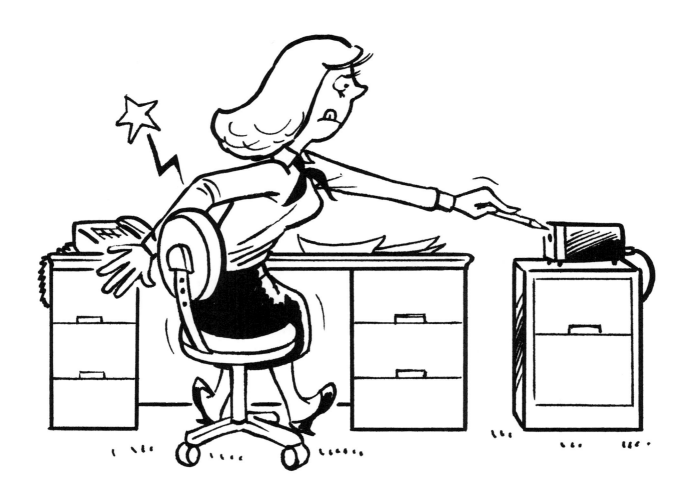

"I heard you need good rotation for golf."

HIP ABDUCTION AND ADDUCTION (MOVEMENT SIDEWAYS)

Self-Test and Exercise for Hip Joint Abduction and Adduction

The purpose of this exercise is to help maintain or improve the range of motion and strength in hip joint motions of abduction (legs apart) and adduction (legs together).

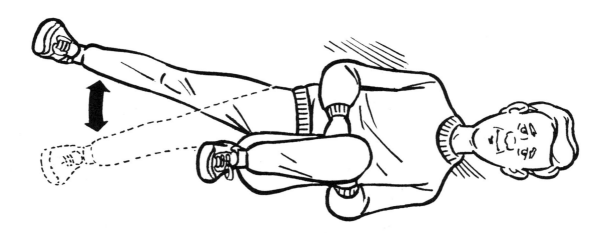

Starting Position: With your left knee to your chest and your right leg out straight, slide your right leg from side to side five times. Return to the starting position. Repeat the exercise with your left leg.

Next, starting with legs out straight, do the exercise with both legs at the same time.

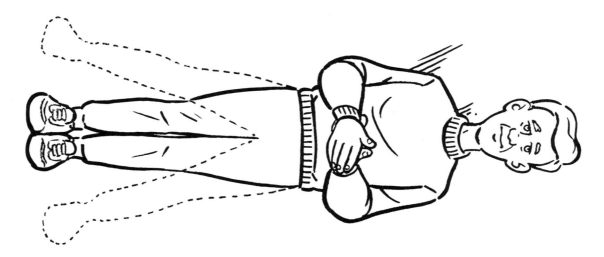

Effect on Golfers

Strength of the hip muscles helps to stabilize your body for good balance during your golf swing. As you shift your weight when you hit the ball, you need strength and flexibility of your hips.

54

The extensor muscles are located along the spine. They move the spine into extension, increasing the arch of the low back, and they straighten the upper back.

Self-Test for Back Extension

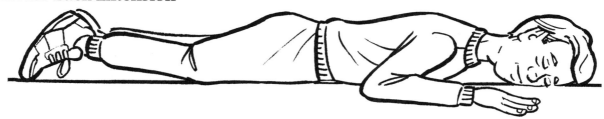

Starting Position: Lie on your abdomen.

Raise your head and shoulders to arch your back; bend your elbows and rest on your forearms. Keep your pelvis flat on the floor to insure that the motion is in the low back. Being able to get into this position as illustrated means you have good back extension.

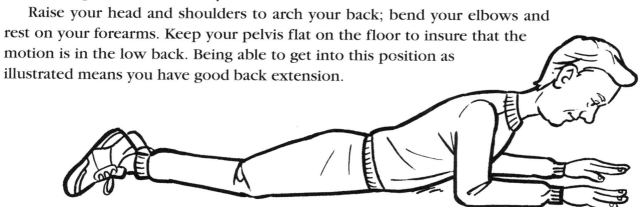

To maintain or improve your flexibility into extension, do the self-test as an exercise. Hold for five seconds. Return to starting position. Repeat ten times.

Effect of Tightness on Golf

Limited ability to straighten your back will also limit your back-swing and follow-through.

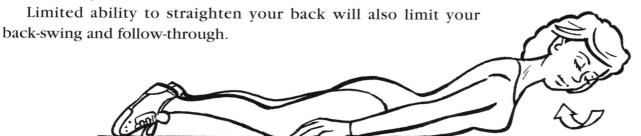

Exercise for Back Extensors

To strengthen your back: Lie on your abdomen with your arms at your sides. Raise your head and shoulders slowly and carefully. Hold for five seconds. Return to starting position and repeat five times. Omit this exercise if there is any discomfort. (You may need to have someone hold your feet down.)

Effect on Golfers

This motion will help your flexibility and strength for your back-swing and follow-through.

LENGTH AND STRENGTH OF SHOULDER MUSCLES

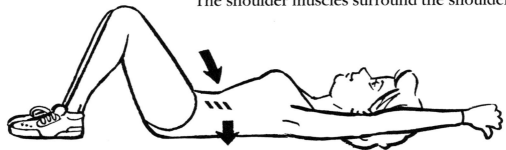

The shoulder muscles surround the shoulder joint.

Self-test for Range of Shoulder Flexion

Lie on your back with your knees bent and your feet resting on the floor. Keep your low back flat on the floor and keep your elbows straight. Raise your arms overhead. Keep your arms close to your head and try to touch them to the floor. If your arms do not touch the floor, you probably have tightness in your shoulder muscles.

Use the test as an exercise to maintain or increase shoulder motion.

Exercise to Strengthen Shoulder Flexors

Note: Omit this exercise if putting your arms overhead causes any tingling in your arms.

Sit on a stool with your back against a wall. Try to keep your back touching the wall and slowly raise your arms forward and up overhead. Hold for five seconds. Then lower arms to your sides. Repeat five times.

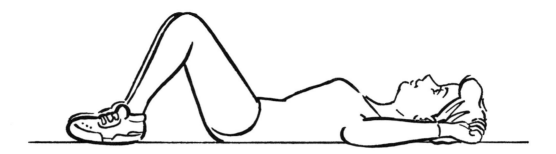

Self-Test for Range of Shoulder Outward Rotation

Keep your low back flat on the floor and place your arms at shoulder level with elbows bent at right angles. Try to touch your forearms to the floor. If your forearms do not touch the floor, you have some limitation of your shoulder outward rotation. As a golfer, you will be limited in your ability to get your right arm outward for your back-swing and your left arm outward for your follow-through.

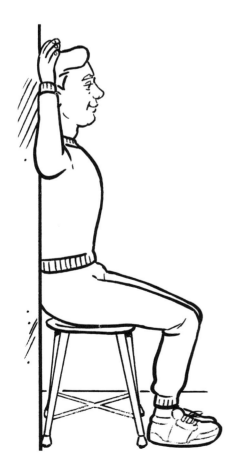

Exercise to Stretch Tight Shoulder Muscles

Use the same positions as in testing. Be sure to keep your back flat, and do gentle stretching. Try to touch your arms to the floor overhead as illustrated above. Stretch for five seconds and return your arms to your sides. Repeat these stretches ten times.

Exercise to Strengthen Shoulder Outward Rotators

Note: Omit this exercise if putting your arms overhead causes any tingling in your arms.

Sit on a stool with your back against a wall. Try to keep your back touching the wall. Start with your arms at your sides. *Slowly* raise your arms sideways to shoulder level. Bend your elbows. Try to press your forearms against the wall. Hold for five seconds. Then lower your arms to your sides. Repeat five times.

TIGHT SHOULDER MUSCLES: EFFECT ON GOLFERS

If your shoulder muscles are tight, you will be limited in raising your arms overhead (A). When attempting to raise your arms as high as you can, the shoulder tightness may cause you to substitute body motion for shoulder motion by arching your low back (B).

Also, if your shoulders are tight when you move your arms across your chest, as in the golf swing, the tightness may cause you to compensate with excessive rotation of your spine in order to achieve the desired motion. (See C below.)

Excessive spine extension and rotation that result from limitation of arm movements can cause significant back problems that may interfere with your golf game.

To Accommodate for Tightness

Accomodate by limiting your backswing and follow-through. You will keep better control of your swing and you will have less chance of hurting your back. (See D below.)

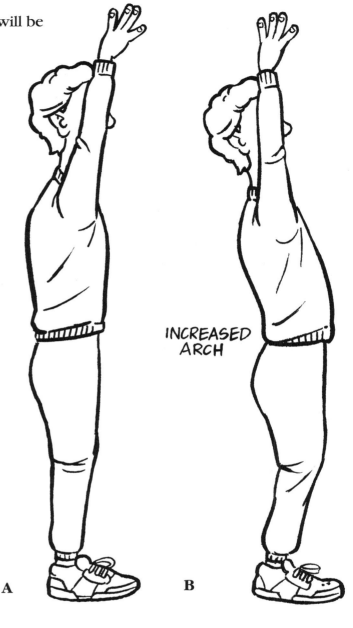

INCREASED ARCH

A   B

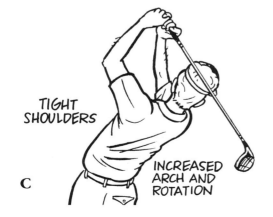

TIGHT SHOULDERS

INCREASED ARCH AND ROTATION

C

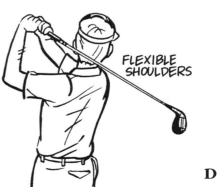

FLEXIBLE SHOULDERS

D

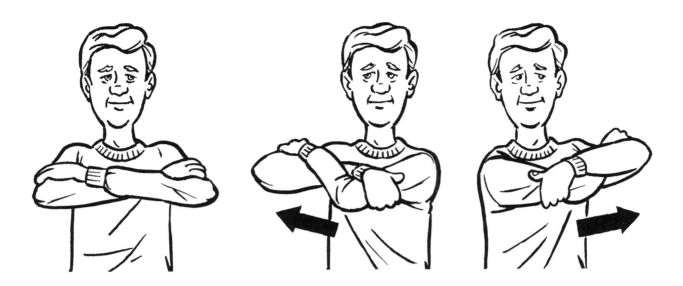

Exercise for Sideways Arm Movement (Horizontal Adduction and Abduction)

Starting Position: Sit on a stool with your back against a wall. Fold your arms at shoulder level as illustrated above.

Stretch the outside of your left shoulder by pulling your left arm toward the right. Hold for five seconds. Then stretch the outside of your right shoulder by pulling your right arm toward the left. Hold for five seconds. Repeat these movements three times. Then lower your arms to your sides.

Exercise to Combine Shoulder Stretch with Neck Rotation

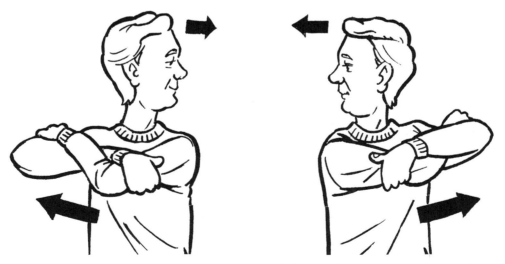

Pull your left elbow across your chest toward the right. Now turn your head to the left and hold this position for five seconds.

Pull your right arm across your chest toward the left. Now turn your head to the right and hold this position for five seconds. Repeat five times to each side.

ROTATION EXERCISES

The following exercises combine hip joint rotation, spine rotation, and shoulder rotation. The exercises should help maintain or improve the rotation movements needed for the golf swing.

Starting Position: Lie on your back with both knees bent and your feet resting on the floor. Use a pillow under your head if needed for comfort (A).

Cross your left knee over your right knee. Your left leg gently pulls your right leg toward the left. This part of the exercise rotates your hips inward (B).

Return to the starting position; do five repetitions *slowly* and *carefully.* Repeat the exercise with right knee over left knee.

The next part of the exercise is for strengthening your rotation (C).

Cross your left knee over your right knee. Your left leg pulls your right leg toward the left (as in B). As you return to the starting position, tighten your abdominal muscles to stabilize your trunk and use your left leg to resist the return motion. Repeat three times to the same side, and then repeat the same exercise with your right knee over your left.

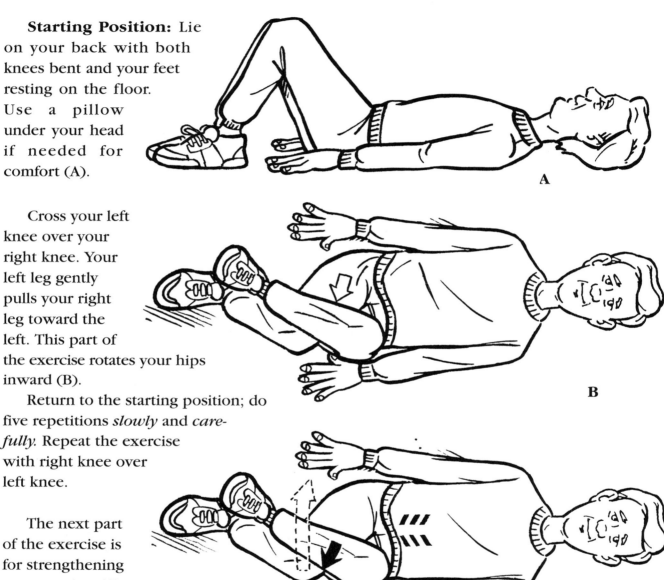

60

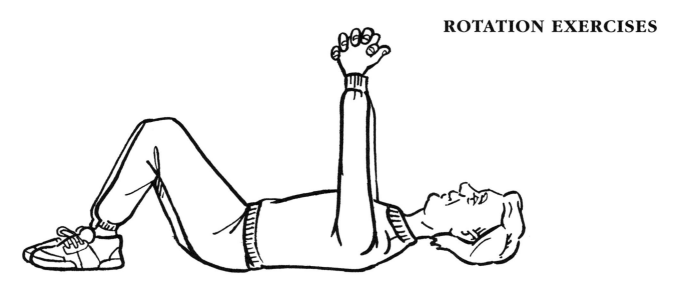

Lie on your back with your knees bent, clasp your hands, and raise both arms directly toward the ceiling.

To stretch across the out- side of the right shoulder, use your left arm to pull your right arm to the left. Return to starting position and repeat. Now do the same on the other side. (Your right arm pulls your left arm to the right).

Start with your knees bent. Do not cross your legs. *Slowly* rotate your legs toward the left as you pull your arms toward the right. Hold for five seconds and return. Repeat the exercise to the same side several times. As your legs rotate to the right, pull your arms to the left. Hold for five seconds and return. Repeat five times.

You can use this exercise to improve your strength by resisting the motion as you return to the starting position.

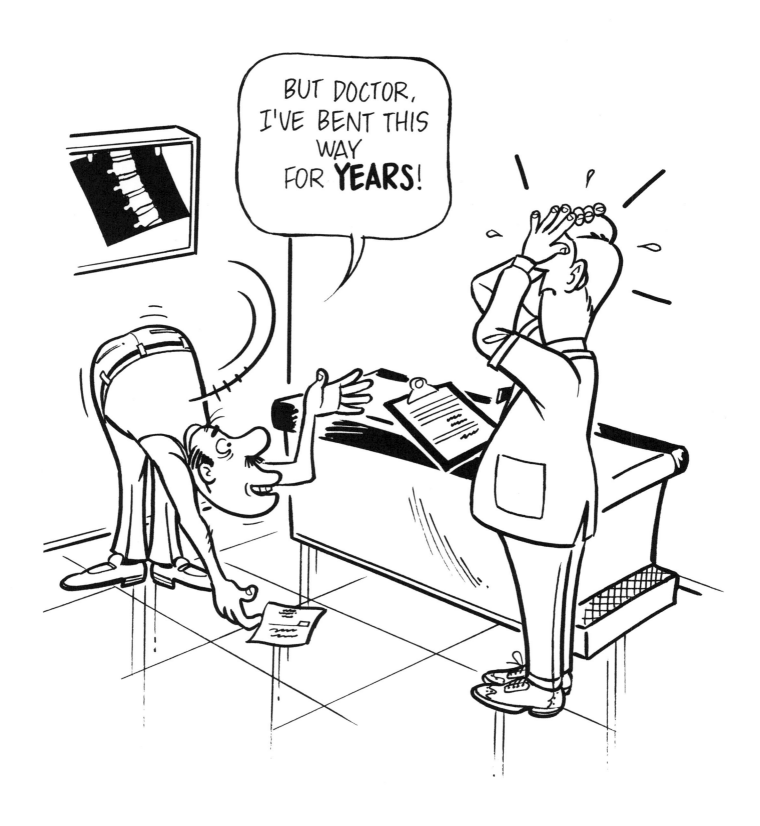

PHENOMENAL ABDOMINALS

The abdominal muscles play a major role in the prevention and management of low back pain because they are important stabilizers of the trunk. For this reason, this chapter is devoted to a detailed but simple explanation about how the abdominal muscles work and how to exercise them properly. These pages may prove to be the most valuable part of the book if you have a low back problem.

Abdominal muscles may be the most mistreated, misunderstood, or neglected muscles in the body, and it is worth your time to try to understand how they function. These muscles should be treated with the same respect that you apply to other muscles. If you put a weight in your hand that is too much for the hand to lift, the muscle is overpowered by the weight and may be stretched and strained by trying to hold it. When exercises put a stretch and a strain on the abdominal muscles, the effect can be harmful.

Abdominal muscles do not attach to the legs, arms, or head. Their only attachments are on the trunk; they can only move the trunk. They can bend the trunk forward, sideways, and rotate it. (Back muscles bend the trunk backward and assist in side-bending and rotation.)

For many years, sit-ups and double-leg raising have been promoted as good exercises to strengthen the abdominal muscles. The fact is that these may be two of the worst exercises you can do if your abdominal muscles are very weak. A review of the next four pages reveals the problems associated with these exercises.

When testing for strength and describing exercises, the abdominal muscles are referred to as "upper" and "lower." These terms are useful in describing the function the muscles perform on the trunk. The upper abdominals act in movements of the upper trunk as in doing a trunk curl (bringing the chest toward the pelvis). The lower abdominals flatten the lower abdomen and act in movement of the lower trunk, as in tilting the pelvis to flatten the low back. (These terms are not meant to imply that there are two separate and distinct upper and lower parts of the abdominal muscles.)

In the following pages, facts are presented to clear up some common misconceptions about abdominal muscles.

MISCONCEPTIONS AND FACTS ABOUT ABDOMINAL MUSCLES

Misconception: Double-leg raising is a good abdominal exercise.

Fact: Abdominal muscles cannot raise the legs because they do not attach to any bone in the leg. Hip flexor muscles raise the legs.

Misconception: If you bend your hips and knees, you can do sit-ups with abdominal muscles.

Fact: The sit-up requires that you bend at the hip joint. Abdominal muscles cannot bend the hip joint because they do not cross over that joint. Hip flexor muscles bend the hip joint.

Misconception: If you bend your hips and knees you will not be using your hip flexors during the sit-up.

Fact: If you did not use your hip flexors you would not do a sit-up at all. The fact is, doing the sit-up with knees and hips bent is a very strong exercise for hip flexors.

Misconception: You have very strong abdominals if you can do repeated sit-ups.

Fact: Many people with very weak abdominals can do repeated sit-ups because the entire movement is done by hip flexors. The weak abdominals cannot curl the trunk so the back arches as the hip flexors raise the body up to a sitting position.

Misconception: Since you can do so many sit-ups, all of your abdominals are strong.

Fact: Even though you have strong upper abdominals and can do many curled-trunk sit-ups, you may have very weak lower abdominals.

Misconception: Both endurance and strength of abdominal muscles can be measured by the number of sit-ups you can do in one minute.

Fact: You may be measuring only the endurance of your hip flexors. If the abdominal muscles are too weak to keep the trunk curled, they may have "endured" only a few sit-ups (or none at all). As you slip into an arched-back position, the hip flexors keep on doing the sit-ups!

Abdominal muscles do not attach to the legs, so they cannot raise the legs. However, abdominal muscles can be affected by the leg-raising exercise. If these muscles are strong, they can hold the back flat during the leg-raising. Strong abdominals will not be hurt by double leg-raising. But if these muscles are very weak, the low back will arch and the abdominal muscles will stretch as the weight of the legs is lifted. As the muscles are strained, they may actually become weaker, and the low back will be subjected to compression and strain. (See pp. 70 -72 for exercises to strengthen lower abdominal muscles.)

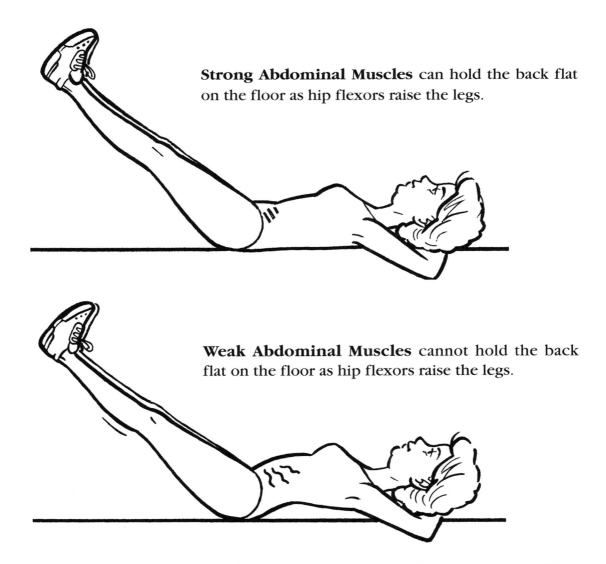

Strong Abdominal Muscles can hold the back flat on the floor as hip flexors raise the legs.

Weak Abdominal Muscles cannot hold the back flat on the floor as hip flexors raise the legs.

Note: Do not use double leg-raising as a self-test for lower abdominal muscles. This is not recommended because it would be difficult to do it accurately without the help of a physical therapist or other trained professional. However, weakness of these muscles is so prevalent that it is a good idea to do the strengthening exercises as a matter of course.

FACTS ABOUT SIT-UPS

The right way to do sit-ups:

First, curl the trunk (flex the spine) by using the abdominal muscles.
Then, use the abdominal muscles to keep the trunk curled as hip flexors perform the sit-up movement.

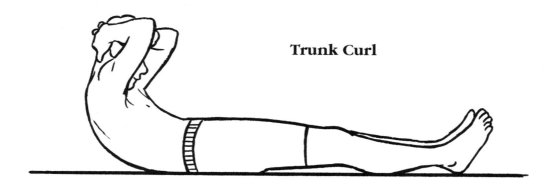

Trunk Curl

Strong abdominals can curl the trunk and that is the only action the abdominal muscles can perform when a person is doing a sit-up exercise. As illustrated above, only the upper part of the body can be lifted up by the abdominal muscles.

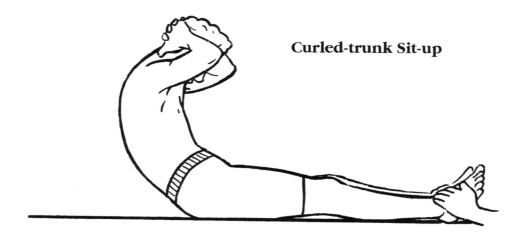

Curled-trunk Sit-up

In order to sit-up, the hip joints must bend. Abdominal muscles do not cross the hip joints, so they cannot assist in the sit-up movement. However, strong abdominal muscles can keep the trunk curled as the hip flexor muscles lift the trunk up to sitting position, as illustrated above.

The wrong way to do sit-ups:

When abdominal muscles are too weak to curl the trunk, the low back will arch as the hip flexors perform the sit-up.

Doing sit-ups this way will *not* strengthen the abdominal muscles. Instead, these muscles will be subjected to stretch and strain, and may be further weakened. Sit-ups with the back arched can also cause compression and strain on the low back.

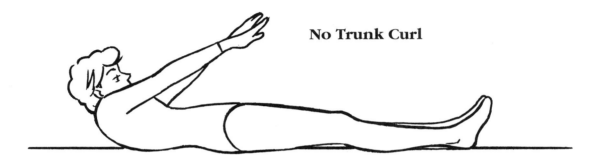

No Trunk Curl

Weak abdominals cannot curl the trunk. The head and shoulders may be lifted slightly as in the figure above. But if the abdominal muscles are very weak, the upper back will not be lifted up at all.

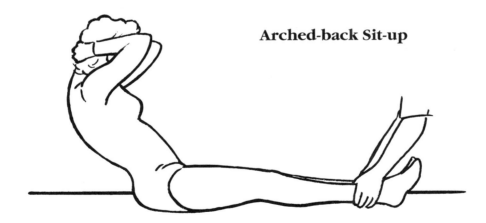

Arched-back Sit-up

When abdominal muscles are too weak to curl the trunk, the sit-up is still performed by hip flexors. However, with the failure of the abdominals to hold the trunk curled, the trunk drops into an arched-back position during the sit-up, resulting in a strain on the abdominal muscles and the low back.

MODIFIED SELF-TEST FOR UPPER ABDOMINAL STRENGTH (TRUNK CURL)

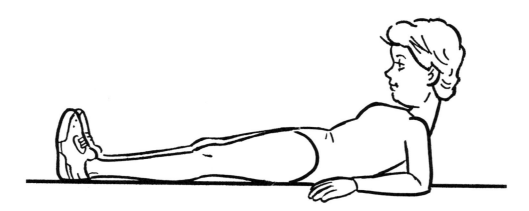

Starting Position: Lie on your back with your legs out straight. Prop yourself up on your forearms as illustrated above. This position will place your spine in flexion (bent forward). The strength of your upper abdominal muscles can then be tested with your arms in three different positions. The object of the test is to find out if you can hold your trunk completely curled without dropping back toward starting position.

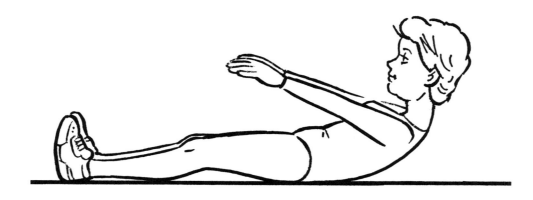

Try to hold the complete curled-trunk position as you take your weight off your forearms, one at a time, and reach forward as illustrated above. Relax back to lying position.

As you take the weight off your forearms, you may find that your legs tend to come up from the floor. (This will happen quite often for men but seldom for women because of the distribution of body weight.) If your feet come up, you may have someone hold them down, but then you must become aware of whether you can still hold your trunk curled. If your back straightens or arches, your abdominal muscles are not holding as they should.

MODIFIED SELF-TEST FOR UPPER ABDOMINAL MUSCLES (TRUNK CURL)

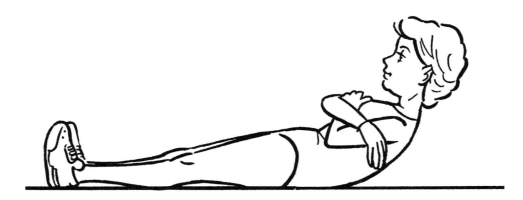

If you were able to keep the trunk curled with your arms in the forward reach position, continue the test as follows.

Prop up on your forearms. Try to hold the complete trunk-curl position as you place your arms across your chest, taking the weight off your forearms one at a time. Relax back to lying position.

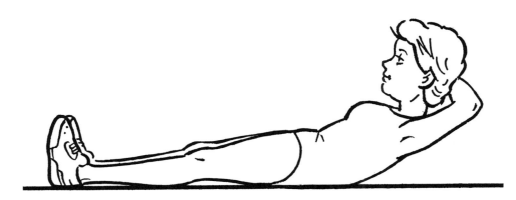

If you were able to keep the trunk curled with your arms folded across your chest, continue the test as follows:

Prop up on your forearms. Try to hold the complete trunk-curled position as you take the weight off your forearms, one at a time, and place your hands behind your head. Relax back to lying position.

Upper Abdominal Exercise (Trunk Curl)

Lie on your back. Tilt your pelvis to flatten your low back on the floor by *pulling up and in with the lower abdominal muscles*. With your arms forward, raise your head and shoulders up from the floor. Do *not* attempt to come to a sitting position, but raise your upper trunk as high as your back will bend. As strength progresses, the arms may be folded across the chest, and later placed behind the head to increase resistance during the exercise.

69

EXERCISES TO STRENGTHEN LOWER ABDOMINAL MUSCLES

Although these strengthening exercises may appear to be "too easy," they are very effective in strengthening the lower abdominals when properly done.

While it is important to do specific exercises to strengthen the abdominal muscles, what really counts is how you correct your posture. In cases of bad posture, the greatest weakness is in the upper back and lower abdomen, and you need to concentrate on trying to hold your upper back straight and your lower abdomen up and in. Doing the lying, sitting, and standing exercises will help you get the feel of good alignment and will help build up the muscle strength where you need it most.

Pelvic Tilt

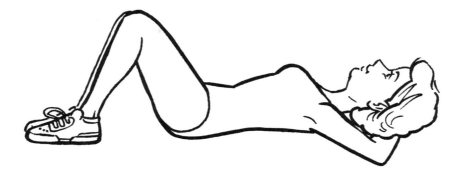

Starting Position: Lie on your back with your knees bent. Place your hands up by your head (or, if that is uncomfortable, leave them resting at your sides). Use a pillow under your head if needed for comfort.

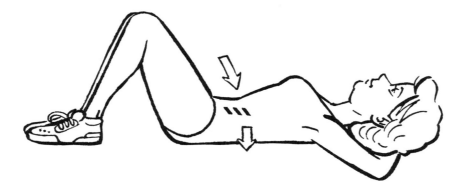

Tilt your pelvis to flatten your low back against the floor by *pulling up and in* with your lower abdominal muscles. Hold for five seconds. Relax and repeat five times. Make the muscles in the lower abdomen very firm. Be sure you do not push with your feet or tighten your buttock muscles to tilt the pelvis — doing so will not strengthen the abdominal muscles!

Heel Slide

This exercise strengthens your lower abdominal muscles if you keep your back flat while you slide your legs.

Starting Position: Lie on your back with both knees bent and your feet resting on the floor. Use a pillow under your head if needed for comfort.

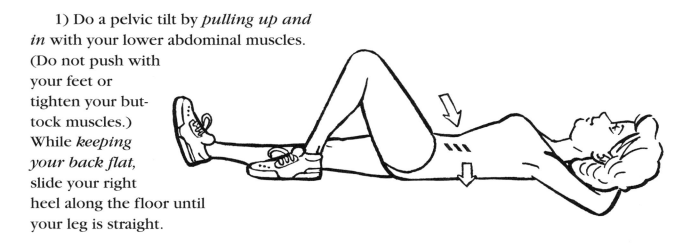

1) Do a pelvic tilt by *pulling up and in* with your lower abdominal muscles. (Do not push with your feet or tighten your buttock muscles.) While *keeping your back flat,* slide your right heel along the floor until your leg is straight.

2) *Keep your back flat* by tightening your lower abdominal muscles as you slide your right leg back to the bent-knee position. Relax, then repeat this exercise with the left leg.

Alternate your right and left legs until you have performed five repetitions on each side. As soon as you are able, you may progress to sliding both legs down at the same time and returning them to the knee-bent position while keeping the low back flat.

EXERCISES TO STRENGTHEN UPPER BACK AND LOWER ABDOMINALS

Note: If you have a problem with tingling in your arms as you raise them overhead, omit raising your arms as you do these wall-sitting and wall-standing exercises. Instead, keep your arms down at your sides with the palms forward as you do the exercises. In standing, heels should be about three inches away from the wall.

The following exercise is done in sitting and standing positions. With your back against a wall, place hands up beside your head. Straighten your upper back. Keep your chin down and press your head back to straighten your neck. (If your upper back is round, *do not tilt* your head back to try to touch the wall.) Hold the position of the head and upper back as you try to flatten your low back against the wall by pulling up and in with the lower abdominal muscles. Keep arms in contact with the wall and slowly move arms to a diagonally overhead position. Hold for a few seconds and then relax, bringing your arms down to your sides. Repeat the exercise five times sitting and five times standing.

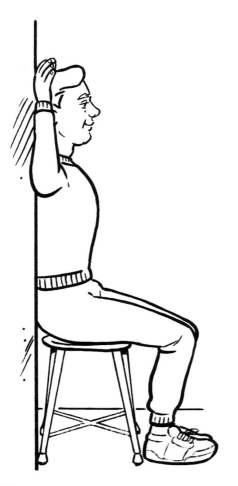
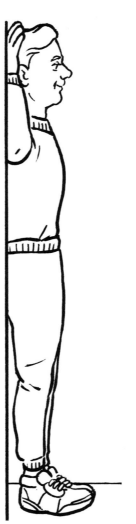
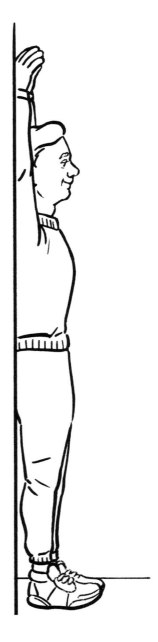

CHAPTER 5

FAIR WAYS TO TREAT YOUR BACK
(Body Mechanics)

Body mechanics refers to the way you use your body in *postural positions* (standing, sitting, or lying) and in *activities* that involve bending, turning, reaching, pulling, pushing, or lifting.

Good alignment provides for good body mechanics. The bones bear weight as they should, and the muscles and ligaments help support the body in proper alignment.

Faulty alignment results in poor body mechanics. The bones are not in the best weight-bearing alignment, and too much strain is thrown on the muscles, ligaments, and joints.

As a golfer, you are subject to the same stresses and strains as anyone else. Whether on or off the course, it is important for you to be able to assume a position of good alignment when standing, sitting, or lying.

The drawings below show both good and faulty postural positions in standing.

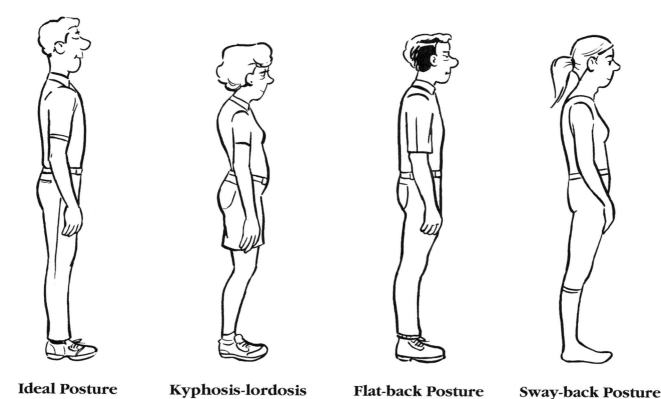

| **Ideal Posture** | **Kyphosis-lordosis Posture** | **Flat-back Posture** | **Sway-back Posture** |

Note: In common usage, sway-back refers to lordosis. In this book, sway-back refers to the specific type of posture illustrated in the right-hand drawing above.

POSTURE IN STANDING

What is your normal standing posture? To see how your body is aligned, stand sideways in front of a full-length mirror and hold a hand mirror so you can see your full reflection from the side.

As you look at your reflection, your ankle bone, the center of your knee, your hip, the middle of your shoulder, and your earlobe should all be in a vertical line.

As a golfer, consider your posture when standing to address the ball, sitting in a golf cart, carrying your golf clubs, and during the golf swing.

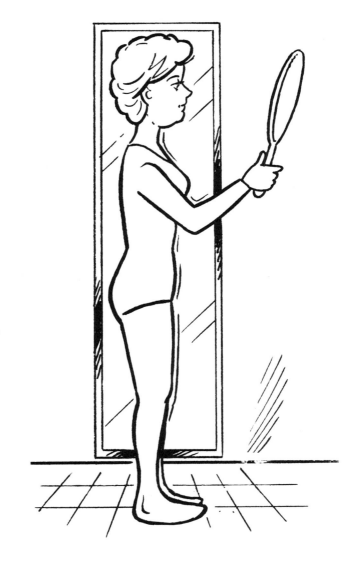

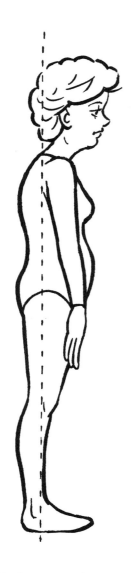

STAND TALL

CORRECT THE
HEAD POSITION BY
STRAIGHTENING THE
UPPER BACK

SQUEEZE
SHOULDER BLADES
TOGETHER AND
PULL THEM
DOWNWARD

FIRM THE LOWER
ABDOMEN

UNLOCK (BUT
DO NOT BEND)
THE
KNEES

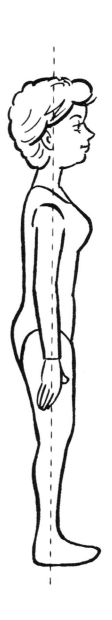

To help you achieve good posture,

1) Stand with your knees in an easy position, neither locked nor bent.

2) Tighten and firm your lower abdominal muscles by pulling the lower abdomen upward and inward.

3) Straighten your upper back by lifting the chest up and forward, but without increasing the arch in your low back. In standing, as the curve in the upper back straightens, the curve in the neck also straightens, and the head assumes a corrected position.

4) Gently squeeze your shoulder blades together, and pull them downward.

POSTURE IN STANDING

**Make your club fit you —
don't change your posture to fit your club!**

Your posture can be affected by the length of your golf clubs. Clubs that are too short will cause you to bend more than you should.

There is more chance of strain if your back is bent too much.

It may be that the length of your club is all right, but that you keep your hips and knees too straight and bend your back too much. You probably need to bend your hips and knees a little more and straighten your back. If you are standing with an excessive arch in your low back, then tighten your lower abdominal muscles to decrease the curve in your low back, and bend your knees slightly.

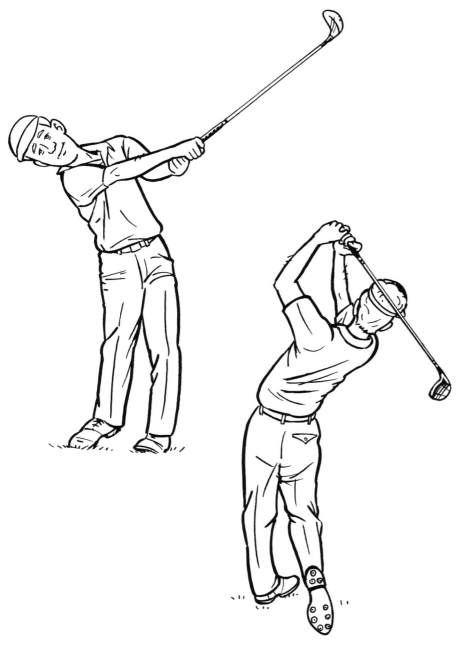

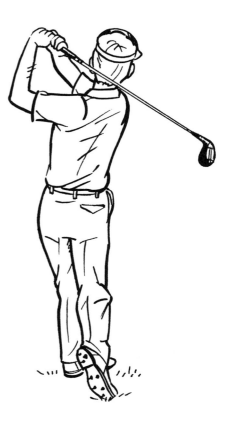

Some important matters to consider about your posture at the end of your golf swing:

1) The amount you bend to the side.

2) The amount you rotate your spine.

3) The amount you arch your spine.

4) The amount of flexibility you have in your shoulders and hips to allow you to rotate to complete your swing.

PUTTING POSTURE

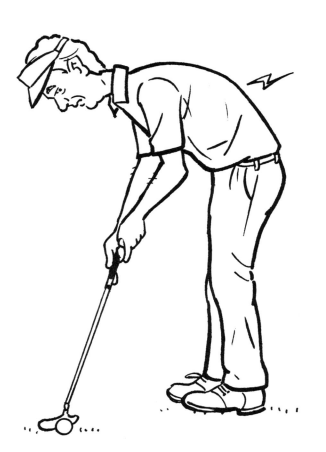

Poor Posture

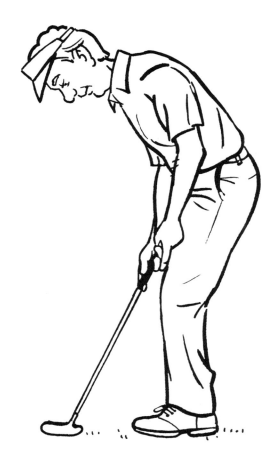

Good Posture

When putting, be aware of your posture. If putting causes you discomfort, then analyze your putting posture in front of a mirror. Is your upper back excessively rounded as you align yourself over the ball? You may be in this position for only a short time so you think it will not affect you, but you repeat this position at every hole.

If your back is excessively rounded, try

1) Straightening your back and bending slightly at your hips and knees to line up your putt.

2) Arching backward as a routine after you putt to counteract your repetitive forward bent posture.

3) Strengthening your upper back with exercises. (See pp. 56, 57 and 72.)

Some golfers have adopted the use of a chest-high putter. This putter permits those golfers to putt in a more upright posture. (See p. 18.)

If you have an "average build" and you have good movement in bending the hip joints and bending the back, you probably are able to stand or sit with your knees straight and bend forward to touch your toes. You probably are able to bend over to place your ball on the tee or pick up your ball without difficulty (A). On the other hand, if your motion in either the back or hip joints is limited, you probably will not be able to do either of these activities without bending your knees (B). (The exercises on pp. 39, 45, and 46 show you how to improve your flexibility.)

Your body build can make a difference in your ability to touch your toes in forward bending. If you have long legs in relation to the rest of your body, you will not touch your toes in forward bending with your knees straight even though you have normal flexibility in your back and hip joints. In this case, if you do stretch to touch your toes, you probably will *overstretch* your back or your hamstrings.

Teenagers who have "shot up" in height, and whose legs have grown long in relation to their trunk, often overstretch the back and/or hamstrings (more often the back) in order to touch their toes.

If, as an adult, you have long legs in relation to your trunk, you are not going to change your build. So when playing golf, you should bend your knees to avoid strain on your back when bending down to place your tee or pick up your ball.

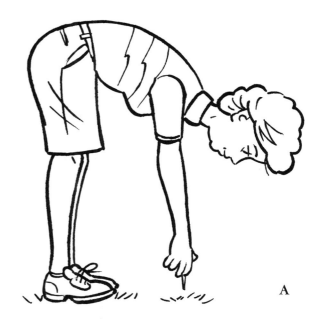

A

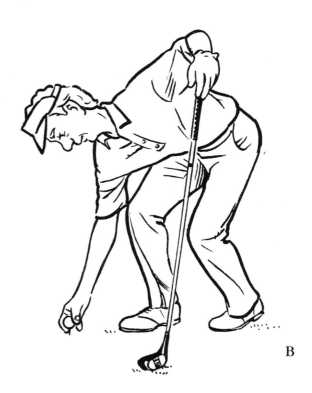

B

BODY MECHANICS WHEN LIFTING

Your body is not meant to be rigid. It is meant to move and continually adapt to moving. Use your body in positions that minimize strain so there is less risk of hurting yourself.

When lifting an object such as your golf clubs, you should follow the guidelines for lifting safely (p. 87).

When getting ready to put your clubs in your car, move other items out of the way to permit you to place the clubs into the car as close to you as possible. Doing so will help protect your back by minimizing the distance you must reach while holding the weight of your golf bag.

When you remove your clubs from the car, do not lean forward and reach or twist.

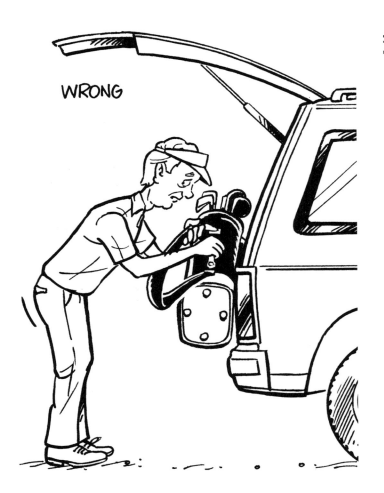

WRONG

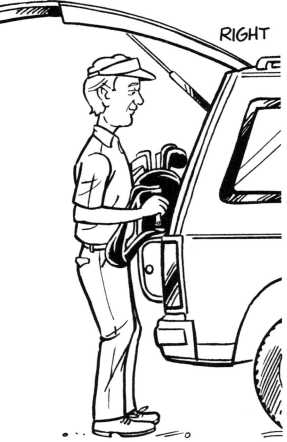

RIGHT

First step close to the car, then pull your clubs close to you and lift them out.

If the back of the car is dirty, it is normal to try to avoid getting your clothes dirty by stepping away. Doing so will cause you to lean forward to reach into the trunk of the car, significantly increasing the strain on your back as you lift your clubs. Instead, have a cloth available to place over the edge of the car to protect your clothes. You then can get close to the car to minimize the strain on your back.

When driving to or from the golf course, you should rest your back against the back of the seat for support. If the seat is too deep from front to back, use a firm cushion behind you. Adjust your car seat if possible, so that your knees are as high as your hips.

Sitting posture is addressed more completely on pp. 88-96.

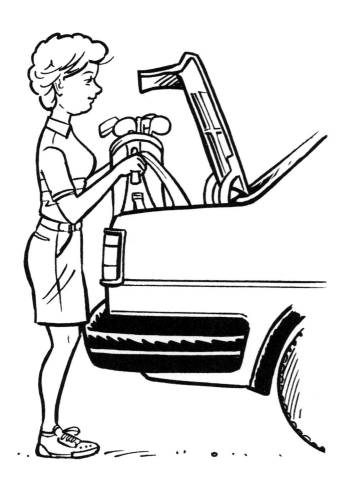

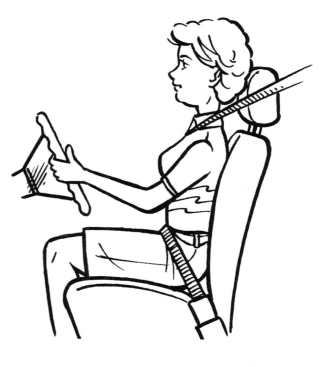

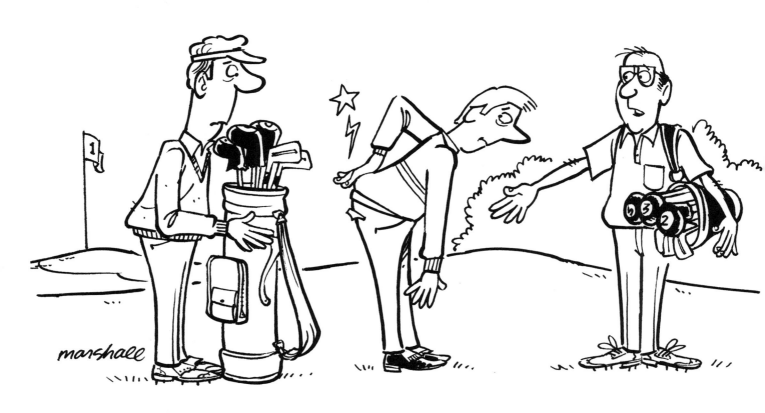

"SORRY, GEORGE CAN'T PLAY GOLF TODAY. HE BENT OVER TO PUT ON HIS SHOES AND HE STILL CAN'T STRAIGHTEN UP!"

BODY MECHANICS WHEN REACHING AND BENDING

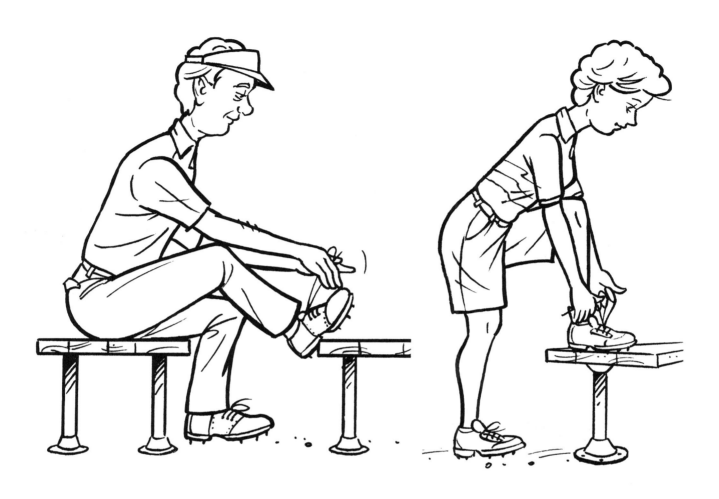

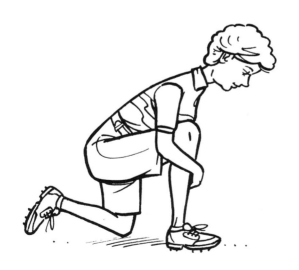

When tying your golf shoes, sitting is the most stable position. If you stand, try placing your foot on some solid support so you do not have to reach and bend too far. If you do not have any trouble with your knees, you may be able to kneel.

BODY MECHANICS WHEN CARRYING GOLF CLUBS

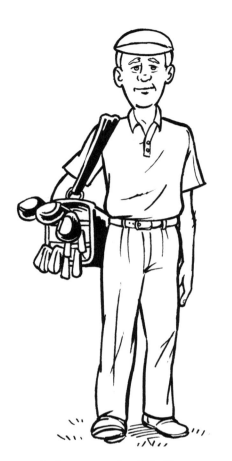

Carry your golf clubs close to your body.

Some golfers increase the stress on their backs by carrying the clubs away from their bodies in order to keep their clothes from getting dirty. If this is a problem, attach a towel to the bag to protect your clothes.

If you usually carry your clubs on the left, occasionally carry them on the right to reduce unequal stress. (Try front nine on the left shoulder, back nine on the right.)

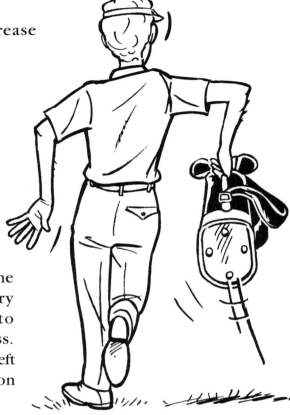

Using a Golf Cart

If the seat is too deep from front to back and you do not get support from the back of the seat, carry a cushion that will fill in the space behind your back.

You need stability for your back while riding in a golf cart. If your back is sensitive to the jarring motion of riding in a cart, you can stabilize your back if you sit tall and firm your abdominal muscles.

Consider wearing a firm elastic back support while you are riding in the cart. Also, you may feel that you have more stability if, instead of being the passenger, you are the driver and can hold onto the steering wheel.

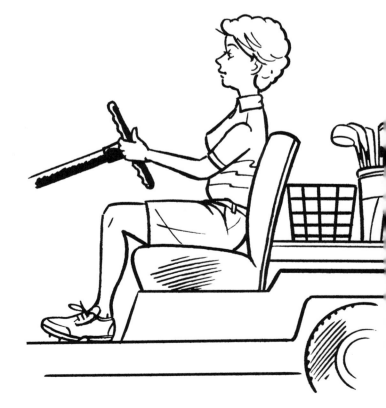

BODY MECHANICS WHEN BENDING AND PULLING

Modified Squat

Golf involves repeated bending. If your back fatigues from too much forward bending, you need to vary the way you bend down. If you are comfortable in a modified squat position, this can be a good alternative.

Using a Pull Cart

When using a pull cart, practice safe body mechanics in order to avoid strain on the shoulders and on the back. Avoid twisting, and keep the cart close to your body — especially when going up or down hills.

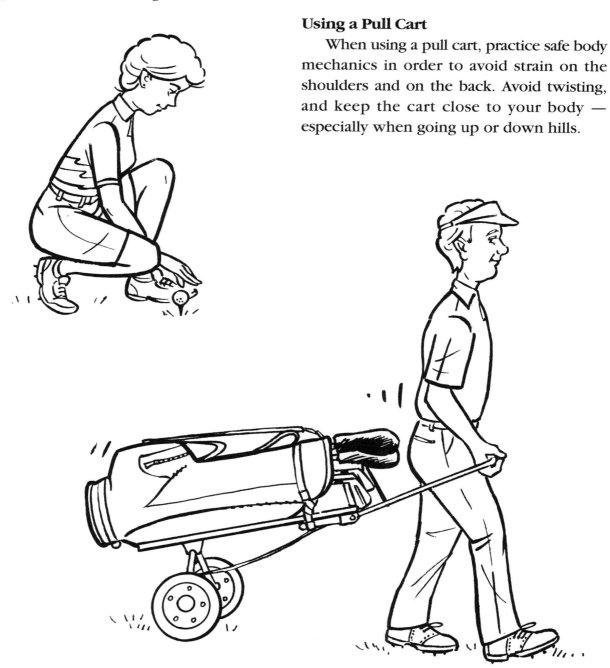

BODY MECHANICS WHEN PUSHING AND PULLING

To keep your body in shape to play golf, use good body mechanics off the golf course as well as on it. Avoid back strain when performing tasks around your house.

For example, when vacuuming the carpet, don't stand in one place and move the cleaner by bending forward, twisting, and stretching as far as your arms can reach.

Instead, keep your body in good postural alignment, hold the cleaner close to you, and walk back and forth, pushing and pulling the cleaner as you go. These same principles apply to such activities as sweeping and mowing the lawn.

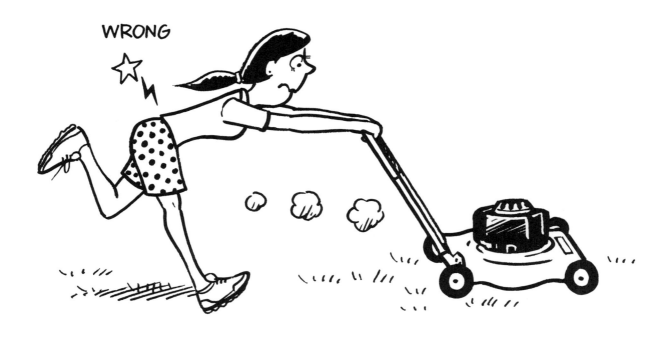

WRONG

Lifting with your body in a bad position or lifting in a wrong way can cause back problems. Here are some ways you can protect your back while lifting:

1) Stand close to the object that you are going to pick up and hold it close to your body.

2) For stability and balance, stand with your feet apart, one foot slightly ahead of the other.

3) Bend your knees slightly.

4 In the forward-bent position, face the object squarely. Avoid twisting your back as you lift the object .

5) Lift the object slowly without jerking.

If your low back has too much flexibility, the illustrations show how you can bend and lift without causing strain of your low back. Stand with your hands on your thighs, your knees bent, and your feet at least shoulder-width apart (somewhat like a baseball player waiting for play to begin).

As you lift the object, your spine is straight. Your bend will occur at your knees and hips. In this position your back muscles will be contracting, and by tightening your abdominal muscles, you will help to stabilize your spine.

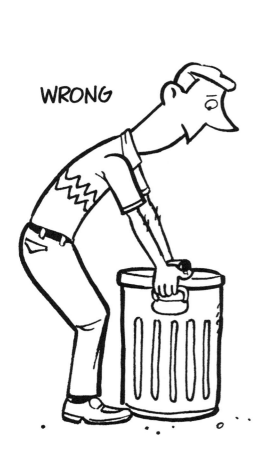

WRONG

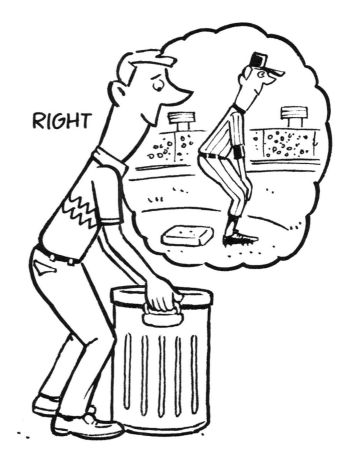

RIGHT

SITTING POSTURE

Many people assume sitting is a position for taking-it-easy-on-the-back. In fact, sitting without proper support to rest against can be very stressful, especially when done for long periods of time.

If you sit up straight (as your teachers used to say), you use muscle power to support your spine in an upright position. Your muscles fatigue and your posture changes as soon as you lose your concentration and relax.

If your chair is a good fit for your body, you can relax, and your back will be supported in good position. (See page 89.)

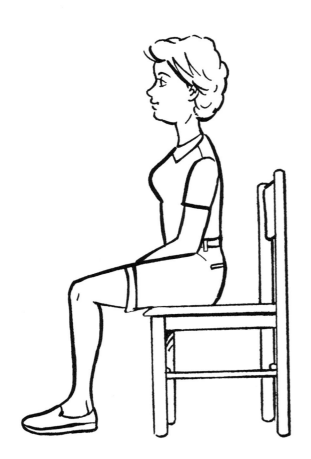

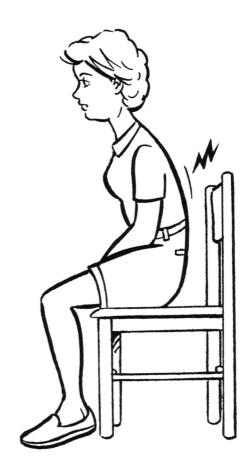

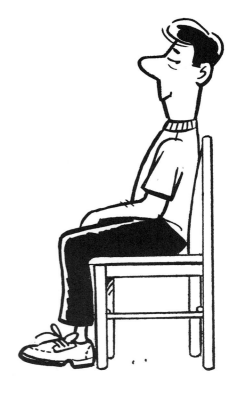

Use the back of the chair for support.

A chair that is a good fit for you must have the seat at the correct height and depth. The back of the chair must support your back, preferably at about a 10° angle. You must sit against the back of the chair to get support.

If the back of your chair reclines, you will distribute the weight of your upper body over a broader area, not just at the base of your spine.

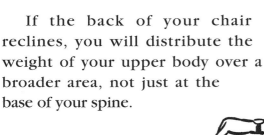

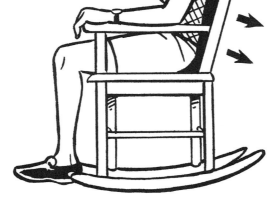

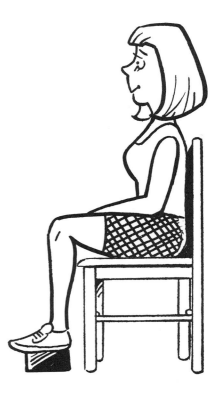

Have your knees as high as your hips or higher.

When you sit with your back against the chair, your feet should be firmly on the floor. If your feet do not touch the floor, you should use a foot rest, either flat or angled, to bring your knees as high as your hips and relieve the pressure on the backs of your thighs.

SUPPORT WHEN THE CHAIR DOESN'T FIT

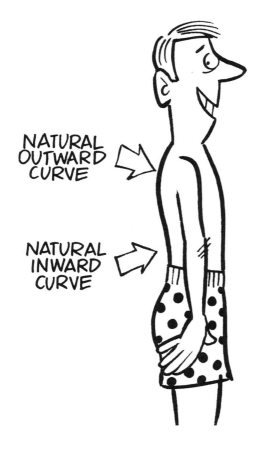

NATURAL
OUTWARD
CURVE

NATURAL
INWARD
CURVE

The natural inward curve in your low back is called the lumbar curve. Some people have an exaggerated inward curve (lordosis); other people have little or no curve (flat back). If the back of the chair does not support your back, then you must use cushions to provide the support. Someone with a lordosis that does not straighten out in sitting may need a cushion behind the low back to fill in the space.

The natural outward curve of your upper back is called the thoracic curve. As one becomes older this curve often becomes more pronounced (kyphosis).

If your upper back curve is prominent, it is very important to fill in the gap below that curve between your low back and the back of the chair so that your entire back has support.

By supporting the entire back, you can avoid excessive pressure over the prominent curves.

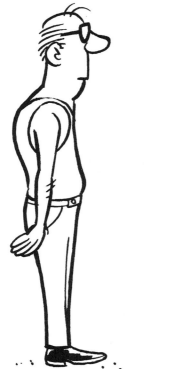

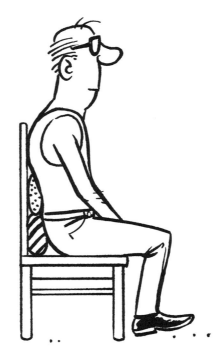

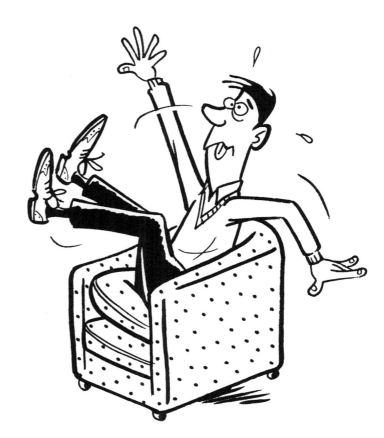

Body shapes and sizes vary, so you cannot expect one chair to fit all people. Some chairs are too soft and some are too straight.

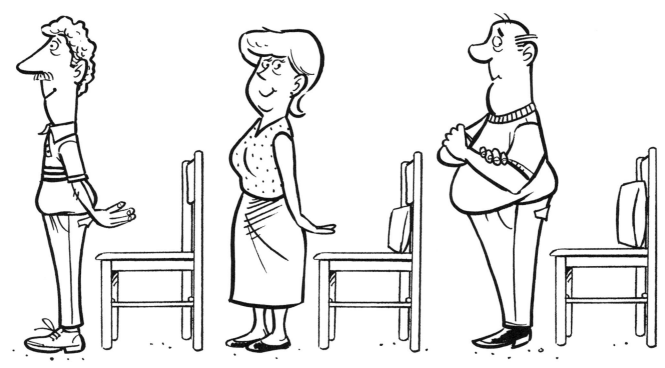

SITTING AT A DESK

Select a chair that permits you to sit close to your work. If the chair has arms which do not fit under the desk, you cannot sit close, and you will be forced to lean forward to reach your work.

A desk chair must be a proper fit for your body and it must be compatible with your desk. You should be able to

1) Sit against the back of your chair with your back properly supported.

2) Place your feet in a comfortable position on the floor or on a foot rest.

3) Position your chair close enough to the desk to permit your body to rest against the back of the chair while your arms are supported on the desk.

4) There must be clearance for your legs when you have positioned yourself at the desk.

A desk chair that has half-arm rests (arm rests that extend from the back of the chair to half of the depth of the seat) is a good choice because it will permit you to position yourself near the desk and still use the arm rest.

Your elbows and forearms should rest comfortably either on the arm rest or on the top of the desk with your shoulders relaxed. If your desk is too high, your shoulders will be raised. If your desk is too low, you will slouch forward.

If the arm rests are too high, your shoulders will be raised and you may develop tension in your neck.

To avoid tilting your head too far forward, you may find it helps to use a slant board to raise and angle your work toward you.

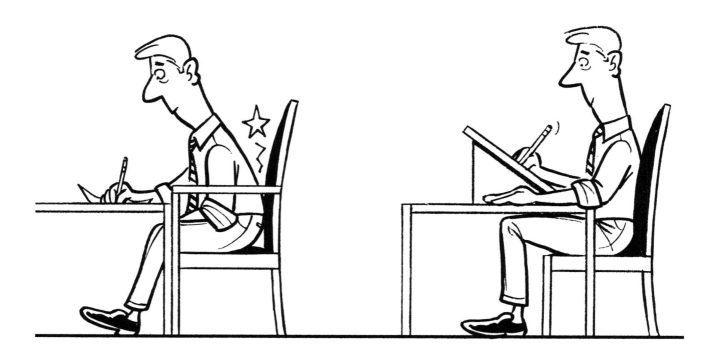

When using a typewriter or computer keyboard, apply the principles described for sitting. You can establish the correct height for your typewriter or computer keyboard as follows:

1) Your back must be resting against your chair and your shoulders should be in a relaxed position.

2) Bend your elbows to an angle of approximately ninety-degrees.

3) Your typewriter or computer keyboard should be at the height that allows your fingers to type with your wrist in a neutral position. The height of your computer monitor should permit your head to be in a level position. Your neck should not be tilted in an uncomfortable position in order to see the monitor.

If you wear glasses with bifocal or trifocal lenses, you will find that you must tilt your head back in order to see through the bottom of your glasses. Doing this for any length of time will put a strain on your neck. The best solution is to get full-lens reading glasses, appropriate for the distance from the computer. It is also important to have good lighting when working at the computer!

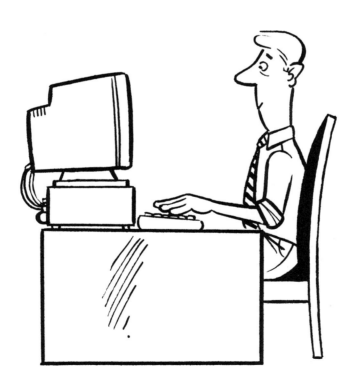

GIVE YOUR BACK A BREAK!

If you are required to sit for long periods of time at work, be sure to stand up occasionally. Keep a pair of walking shoes at your desk, and, if possible, use part of your lunch time to take a walk.

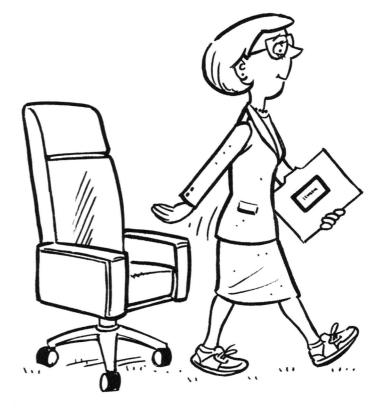

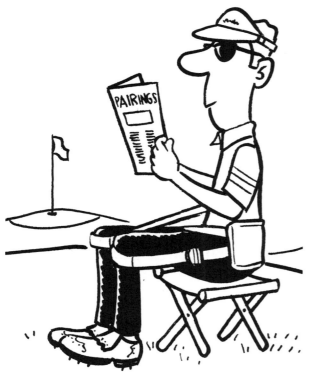

When sitting on a bench or on stadium bleachers, the back is without any support. A type of support that is easy to carry and easy to put on is shown in the illustration at left. The sling-like device has a pad in back which is held in place by straps around the knees and is used to help relieve strain on the low back.

Wear your seat belt!

A car seat is essentially a chair for driving. It must contour to fit your back. If the seat does not fit your back, then use cushions to provide the support where you need it. If your car has a bucket seat which tends to be rounded, the support that you require will be different from that required for a straight bench seat.

Sitting in a bucket seat for an extended period of time without correct back support may make it difficult for you to straighten up as you get out of the car. If this is a problem for you, try using a cushion behind your back or on the seat. An arm rest will permit some relaxation for your shoulders and neck.

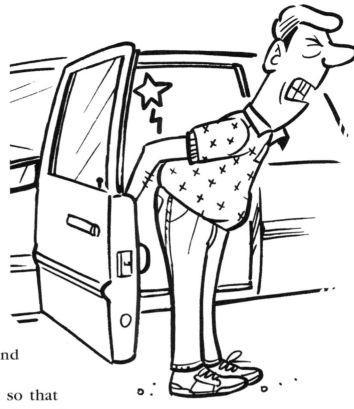

Position your body on the car seat so that you do not have to reach for the pedals or the steering wheel. If you move your seat to the maximum forward position and you still cannot reach the pedals or steering wheel, you need to place a cushion behind you.

A person of average height can make adjustments to car seats, but a tall person does not have that option. If you are tall, you need to avoid driving a car that forces you to slump down in order to see through the windshield. The bad position of the head and neck puts you at risk of strain or injury. Choosing the right car can be an important matter for you.

SITTING ON A PLANE

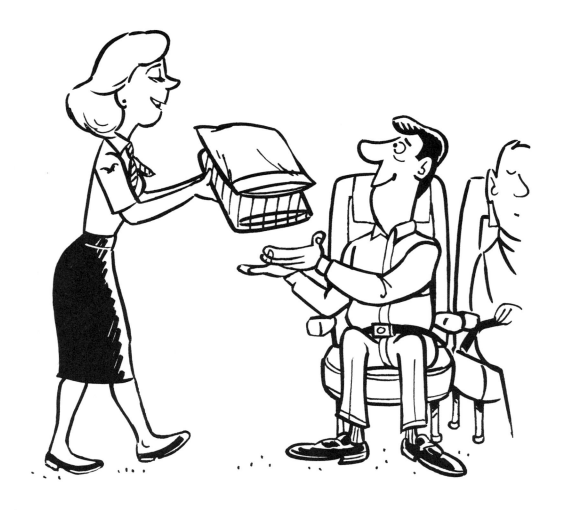

Some airline seats look like they were made for a very tall person with round shoulders and a forward head! The seat forces you into a rounded-back, forward-head position. If you have been "crunched" into a seat like that, you need to make some adjustments.

Ask the stewardess for a pillow and a blanket. Fold the blanket to make a pad that fills in the hollow in the seat back. If your head is still pushed forward, add more padding by using a pillow in addition to the folded blanket.

If you can get yourself into a comfortable position, you can "sit back and enjoy the flight" — unless, of course, you are on a long flight and you develop aches and pains from sitting still. Then you may need to stand up and walk up and down the aisle occasionally.

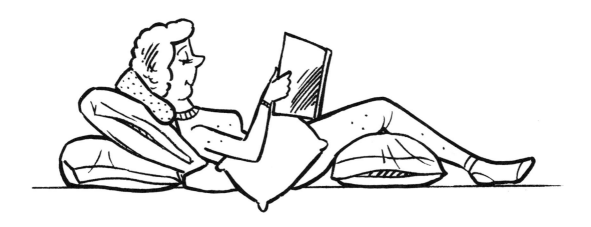

Sleeping Positions

When you are away from home for work or for a golf vacation, be sure your back is supported when you sleep. You may need to make some accommodations in order to get good back support. Sometimes the solution is to put the mattress on the floor. Sometimes you can get comfortable just by using extra pillows to provide support where you need it. (See pp. 106-108.)

Reading in Bed With Your Head Propped Up

Reading in bed can be a "pain in the neck" unless you have your body and your book in good positions. Having your neck bent forward too much is not good. Having your neck bent backwards by tilting your head back (as you are bound to do if you are wearing bifocals) is not good either!

To position your body, you need to get into a partial sitting position with your head, upper back, and

low back well supported. Then you need to have your book held or propped up at a level for your easy reading. If you are holding the book, put pillows under your arms for support. You may be able to avoid holding the book by propping it up on a slanted board held in place by pillows.

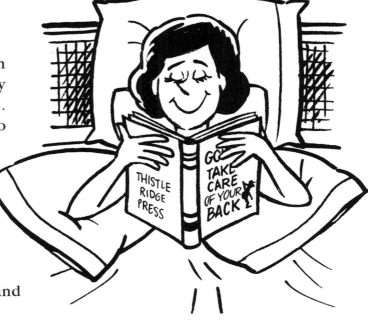

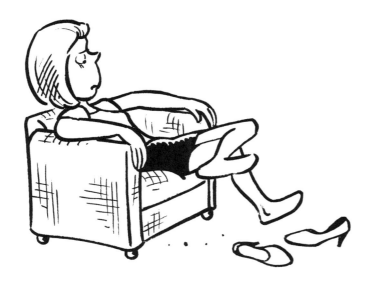

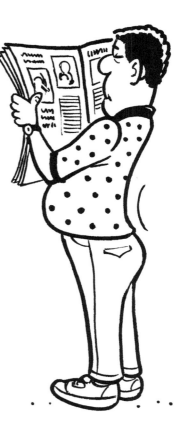

"Why Does
My Back Hurt
So Much?"

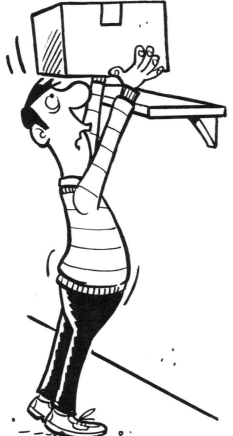

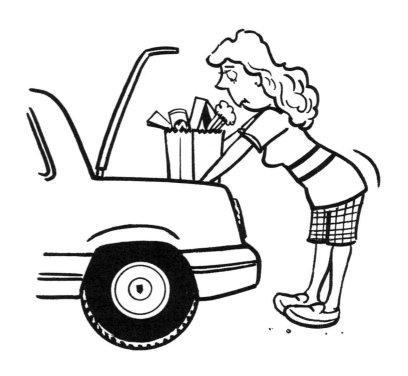

BIG BACK ATTACK
(What to Do If You Hurt Your Back)

Back pain is almost as common as the "common cold." Just as a cold may be as slight as a "sniffle," back pain may be just annoying, or it may be severe enough to keep you off the golf course.

Back pain may "come and go" or it may be constant. The discomfort or pain may be present only in the morning, or it may hit you more at the end of the day. It may come on gradually or suddenly; it may last a few days or a long time. It may affect you while you play golf or it may come on after the round. Back pain may be something you put up with because it does not interfere with your rest or your activities. However, it may be severe enough to put you flat on your back.

If you have a sudden attack of back pain — a big back attack — *don't panic!* Take comfort in the statement that most people who develop back problems get better in about two weeks.

Many factors enter into making decisions about immediate care for someone who has an acute attack of back pain. First, recognize that you need help. As in any emergency, you need to get help from the people who are there with you.

An acute attack that seems to have come on suddenly, perhaps caused by a faulty or stressful movement, may be a strain of muscle, or a sprain of ligament or joint — none of which is trivial, but which, if handled properly, should heal.

Do not adopt the attitude that you will get better if you force yourself to carry on in spite of the pain. If you are on a golf course when the pain occurs, let people help you. Try using your golf club as a cane if doing so helps you move with less pain. Don't take chances. Even one more swing can make the pain worse.

If you get a shooting pain down the leg, you must stop playing, but *don't panic.* Your first thought may be that you have "slipped a disc" (herniated a disc). But like muscle strain or ligament sprain, most disc problems are resolved by conservative measures. These measures consist mainly of restricted activities, bed **rest** if needed, **ice,** heat or medication to relieve pain, back **supports,** and **exercises** to help prevent recurrences. Not every slipped disc requires an operation; less than five percent go to surgery.

You are highly motivated to get well, and in a hurry. That's fine. Such motivation is important for recovery, but be sensible.

CAUSES OF BACK PAIN

Many people have been told they just have to learn to live with low back pain. Do not adopt that attitude without learning about some of the simple, effective ways in which you can help yourself. Improving your posture, strengthening muscles that are weak, and stretching those that are tight can make a big difference in how you feel. For you, as a golfer, the difference may mean playing without injury and even improving your game. If back pain keeps you from playing golf, the information in this chapter can be useful in helping you to return.

Common Causes of Back Pain

There are many factors that contribute to a person's having back pain. These include lack of flexibility, excessive flexibility (causing instability), lack of strength or endurance, repetitive injury (often referred to as cumulative trauma or overuse injury), staying in one position for a prolonged time (causing fatigue), faulty posture (usually the result of one or more of the other causes listed) and trauma.

These contributing factors may be associated with any of the following:

1) Problems of the muscles, tendons, ligaments — tears, sprains, and strains.

2) Problems of the joints — degenerative changes, irritation, inflammation.

3) Problems of the discs — degenerative changes, narrowing of disc space, bulging discs, or ruptured (herniated) discs.

4) Problems of the nerves — pinched, irritated.

Other Causes

However, it is also important to alert you to conditions other than the common ones that may cause back pain. These include rheumatoid arthritis, osteoporosis, spine fractures, infections of the bones and the discs, spinal stenosis, and conditions of organs (such as the kidneys) and vessels (such as the aorta). Cancer of the spine or adjacent organs can also present itself as back pain. If low back pain does not seem to improve in a matter of a few weeks, there should be an examination by a physician to rule out more serious causes. You should be aware that a condition such as osteoporosis (loss of bone mass) may be the cause of a fracture in the back or of the hip which can occur by an otherwise ordinary turning or bending motion.

If a pain radiates into your leg or you lose muscle strength in your leg or foot, you should consult your doctor. If your back problem causes you to lose control of your bowel or bladder you should seek immediate emergency care.

Everyone who has a back problem wants to be cured. However, back pain can, and often does, recur. Unless you do something to correct the problem, each episode tends to last longer than the previous one, and episodes may recur more frequently.

Lack of Flexibility

Lack of flexibility results in restricted range of motion, and usually, muscle tightness. When restricted motion exists in one joint, it often results in excessive range (instability) of other joints in an attempt to compensate for the tightness elsewhere.

Lack of Strength or Endurance

Lack of strength or endurance can also cause instability and strain on joints. (See abdominals, Chapter 4, and hip and knee extensors, p. 40.)

Repetitive Use Injury

Motions that occur repeatedly in one direction can eventually lead to painful conditions or over-use injuries.

Imbalance of strength or flexibility may result from excessive repetitive motion, whether the motion involves bending, arching backward, side bending, or rotating. Repetitive motion occurs in golf because the more forceful movement always occurs in the direction in which you hit the ball. Become aware of other motions you do repetitively and try to alter your routine. *When practicing, occasionally swing your golf club in the opposite direction from your normal swing,* and at times, do this with a weighted club.

Prolonged Positions

Your back may function well in one position, but if it remains in that position for too long it may become stressed. A change in position may lessen or relieve the strain entirely. For example, if you, as a golfer, practice putting for a long time and have trouble straightening up after bending forward, you may get relief by standing up and arching backward after several putts.

Or, when practicing putting, use only three balls at a time to putt. This forces you to change your position by standing up and walking to retrieve the balls.

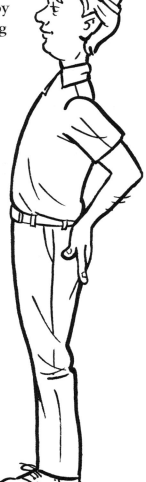

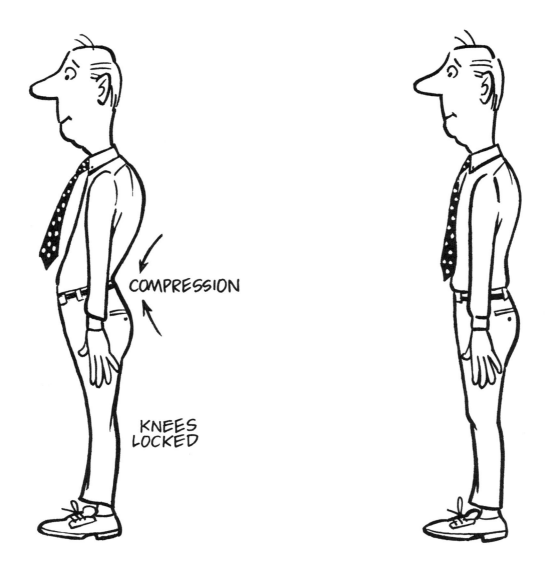

Poor Posture (Prolonged Compression or Prolonged Stretch)

Can bad posture cause or increase back pain? Yes it can!

You may have too much arch in your low back causing the joints to be compressed. The increased arch in your low back is often caused by tight hip flexors. (See p. 43.) This posture may eventually cause sufficient strain to produce pain. You can help change your posture and decrease the arch in your low back by stretching your hip flexors, and strengthening your lower abdominal muscles to provide support to your back.

A locked (back-knee) position also contributes to bad posture of the back, tending to increase the arch. Avoid the "locked" position. Stand with the knees "easy" but not bent.

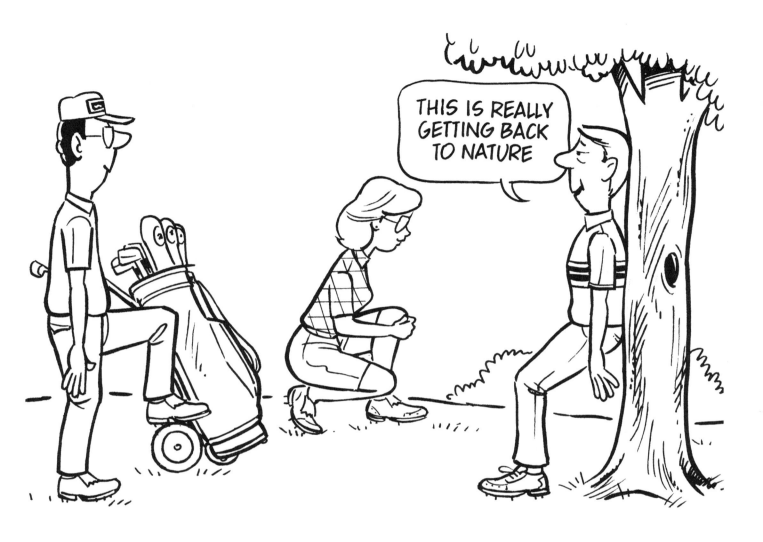

If your low back aches because it has too much forward arch (lordosis), the following suggestions can help reduce the discomfort:

1) Firm your lower abdominal muscles to level your pelvis.

2) Place one foot forward on an object that is about six to eight inches high.

3) Lower your body into a squat position (provided you have no problems with your knees).

4) Sit down and bend forward.

5) Lean your back against a wall or a tree.

These positions can reduce the arch in your low back and help relieve the symptoms.

STANDING POSTURE

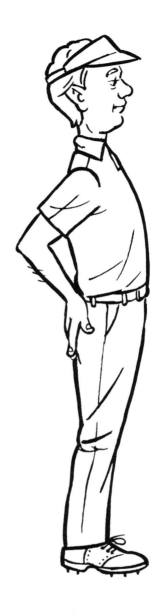

Pain may be caused by excessive rounding of your upper back and a forward head.

The forward head position does not permit full rotation of the neck. This will have an effect on your neck motion in your golf swing. (See pp. 4, 12, and 30.) Good postural alignment of your head will enhance your ability to rotate your head.

To improve this posture, straighten your upper back. As you straighten your upper back, your head will assume a good position with your ear lobe in line with your shoulder. (See p. 74 and 75.)

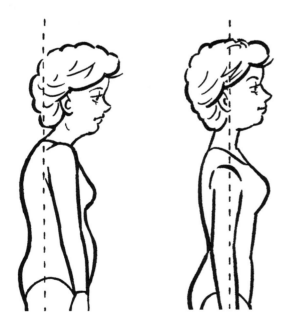

If you must stand or sit in a forward-bent position for long periods of time, you may feel stiff when you try to straighten up. While in a standing position, place your hands on your back and gently bend backward to increase your flexibility. You may also try to do the back extension exercises to help maintain your natural curve.

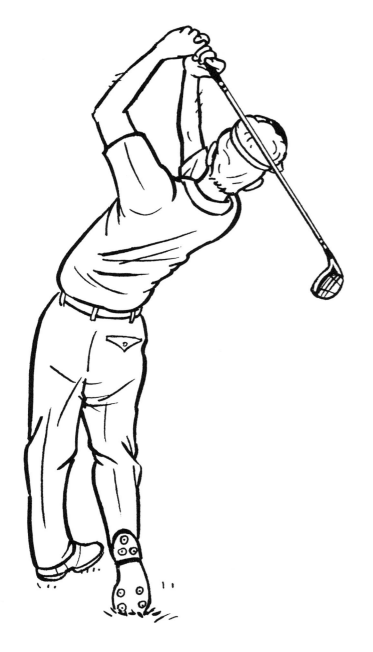

It may stress a bone causing a fracture, or it may cause an impact injury that compresses a joint or pinches a nerve.

In golf, trauma could result from something as simple as over-swinging into a slope, or over-swinging into your follow-through (excessive rotation and arching with side-bend), causing stress to the joints of your back by over-compressing them.

An imbalance in strength may predispose to trauma. The golf swing is conducive to muscle imbalance because the more forceful movement is in the direction that you hit the ball. Therefore you must work at strengthening the opposing muscles. As a routine when you practice, swing a weighted club in the opposite direction from your natural swing.

Avoid preventable back injuries when possible:

1) Wear your seat belt.

2) Be sure throw rugs are securely attached to the floor.

3) Do not leave electric cords or objects in the path of travel.

4) Wear good shoes for walking.

5) Use a hand rail when climbing or descending stairs.

6) Stay as fit as possible to avoid injury.

Trauma may be caused by something as severe as falling, or as simple as slipping on wet grass and lurching to catch your balance.

Trauma to your back may result from a jarring or vibrating motion, from lifting an object that is too heavy for you, or from an accident. The trauma may cause a muscle strain, a ligament sprain, or a tendon tear.

Since all back pain or acute attacks of back pain are not alike, it is impossible to make suggestions that will cover all possibilities. This book is not a substitute for seeking medical attention when you have a back problem, but these suggestions may help you in your recovery process.

As a general rule, go slowly and progress gradually. Stop activities or change positions that cause pain. Err on the side of caution. It is better to prevent a recurrence than to be off the golf course for a longer time.

Sports medicine often refers to first aid as R-I-C-E (Rest, Ice/Heat, Compression, Elevation). Insofar as some back pain resembles a sports injury, R-I-S-E (Rest, Ice/Heat, Support, Exercise) can be applied.

Rest

Getting Into and Out of Bed

If you you have had an attack of back pain and you are more comfortable at bed rest for the first day or two, you may find that getting into and out of bed may be painful.

When you are ready to lie down, sit on the side of the bed, support yourself with the arm on the side toward the head of the bed. Holding your back straight, and keeping your hips and knees bent, let yourself down sideways by gradually bending the elbow until you rest on your forearm. Keeping the hips and knees bent, gradually bring your legs up onto the bed as you lie down. From that position, you may roll onto your back or onto the other side. Roll over, moving your whole body as a unit. When you get out of bed, reverse the process.

Frequently patients with back injuries have muscle relaxants or anti-inflammatory medications prescribed. You can maximize effects of the medicine by learning how to support your body and relax more easily. The following positions will show you how to use pillows and cushions for support.

Lying on your Side

If you lie on your side on a sagging cushion or mattress, your body will sag down at your waist. This position is the same as if your spine were bending sideways. Lie on a firm surface that will support your spine. Try placing a small cushion under your waist to allow your spine to rest in neutral position.

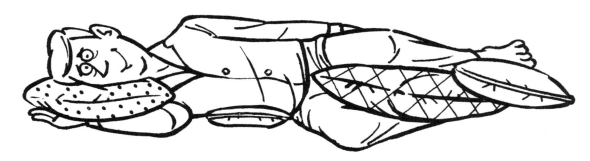

When the surface you rest on matches the contours of your body and holds you in a comfortable position, you can relax. All too often the couch or bed does not give enough support to your spine. The use of pillows and cushions can help compensate for the lack of support.

Support your head with pillows so that it is not raised too high or dropped too low. Place a small cushion or folded sweat shirt under your waist. Place two pillows between your legs — one between your thighs and one to support the calf and foot of the top leg. Another pillow should be tucked in front of your abdomen if you tend to roll forward or behind your back if you tend to roll backward.

When you support yourself with pillows, your body can relax and be held in a comfortable position. Without the pillows for support you tend to stiffen your body to brace yourself from pain.

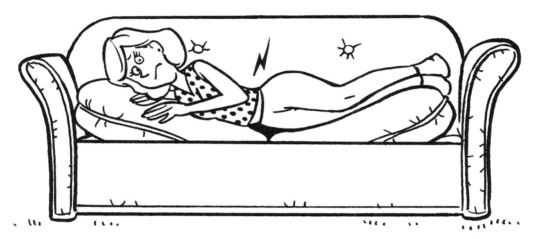

Soft, sagging cushions do not help a painful back.

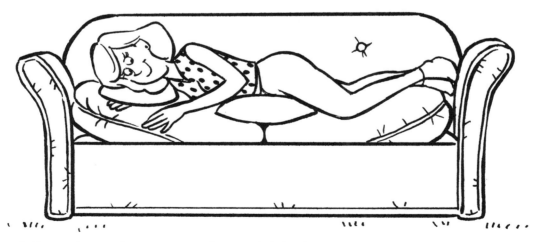

If there is no firmer couch available, build support with pillows to make yourself as comfortable as possible.

Lying on your Back

1) Place a pillow under your head. For additional comfort, tie a shoelace or a string around the center of a soft pillow to convert it into the shape of a butterfly. Contour this pillow under your head and around the sides of your neck.

2) Place one or two pillows under your knees. If you want to achieve additional relaxation, use pillows to support your arms.

3) Your mattress should be firm and not sag under your body weight. Your boxspring should be very firm. If it is not, use a 3/4" plywood bed board under the mattress.

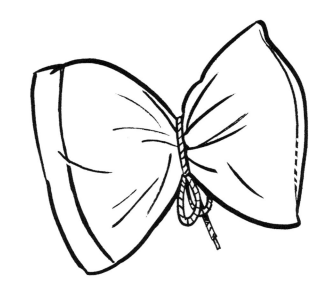

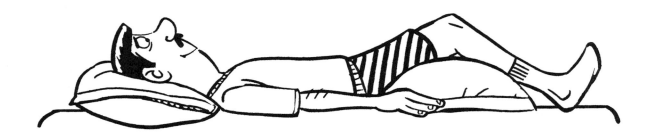

Another position, when lying on your back, is to support your legs in the "90/90" position. Lie on your back with your knees resting on enough pillows to support your hips and knees at approximately a ninety-degree angle. This position permits your spine to rest flat with your legs completely supported. If your back does not relax against the bed, you may want to try a small towel roll under your back if some pressure against your spine eases your pain.

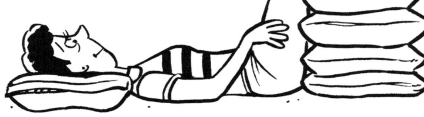

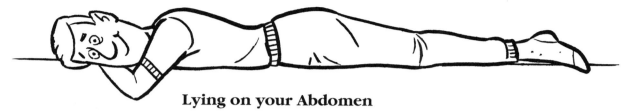

Lying on your Abdomen

You may have heard the advice that you should never lie on your abdomen when you have a back problem. However, there may be times when lying on your abdomen or being propped up on your elbows will provide the best relief for back symptoms.

If pain results from excessive arching of the low back, lying on your abdomen probably will be uncomfortable for you; if it increases or causes your pain to spread into your buttock or leg, you should not continue to lie in this position.

If you hurt your back by bending forward, then do not try to rest by slouching on a couch or sitting in a chair without proper back support. These positions are too similar to the bending position in which you hurt yourself. You may be able to sit comfortably if you support your back in a straight position.

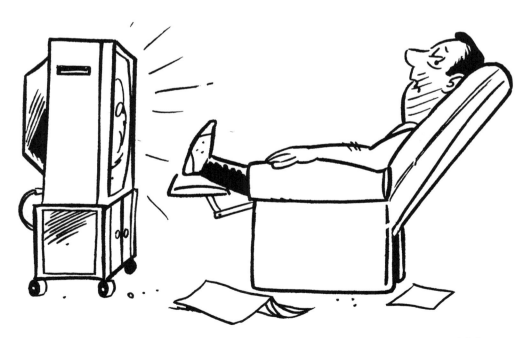

Ice Packs

Icing your back often helps relieve pain.

One method of icing is to make an ice pack. Place about two dozen ice cubes or an equivalent amount of crushed ice in a plastic bag, and *wrap securely in a towel.* Place the ice pack and towel on your back for a few minutes at a time if it helps relieve your pain.

A quick and clever substitute for an ice pack is a bag of frozen peas.

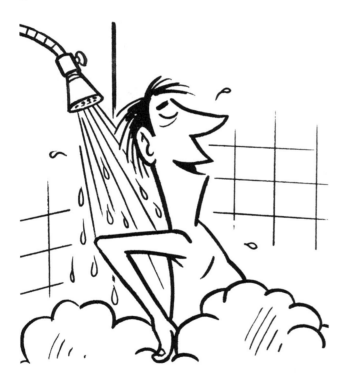

Heat

For some people, heat works better than ice for relaxation and reduction of pain. Try warm tub baths or showers, or moist heat packs. The heat should be comfortably warm, but *never* hot enough to burn your skin.

Either ice or heat may be used several times a day. Choose whichever one is most effective for relieving your symptoms.

R-I-S-E: Back Supports

The purpose of a spinal support or brace is to hold your spine in a comfortable and protected position until movement can occur without pain. A support may be a girdle, an over-the-counter athletic wrap, a firm band (like a wide belt), or a corset or brace fitted by a specialist.

If you are in a situation where you can "wait and see" if you get better or worse, then the following information may be a big help to you.

Your back muscles may be in spasm, and you can't move your back in any direction. You really are in pain. You must realize that sometimes the spasm is nature's way of keeping you from moving so you will not injure yourself further. When the muscles have to hold you rigid, the pain does not go away. Many times you can get relief if you can put on a support that keeps you from moving your body. If the muscles are relieved of the burden of support, they tend to relax and your pain diminishes. At the same time, you have assurance that the support will help protect you from moving in a way that will cause further injury.

If a support helps you when you are up, you may find that it also helps to keep it on while lying down.

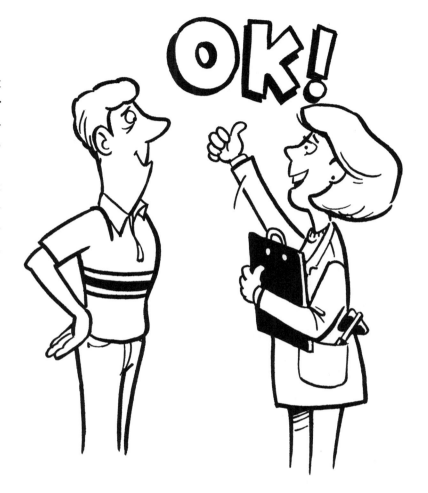

(Support, continued)

But how do you get a support in a hurry? Ask your doctor or physical therapist for a recommendation about where to go to get an appropriate support.

Sometimes a support does not help. It may hold you in a position that is painful. Do not continue to use it if it makes you worse.

Some people worry that once you wear a support, the muscles will get weaker. However, the strain on the weak muscle may be the reason for the pain. The support relieves the strain and the muscles have the chance to function more normally and improve their condition.

R-I-S-E: Exercise

Sometimes walking will actually help to decrease pain. However, you must stop walking if your symptoms increase.

If your pain increases when you sit, you probably will try to avoid sitting. If you must sit, try to sit in the proper position as described on p. 89.

When you begin to feel ready to play golf and have your physician's approval, start with exercises and a walking program.

Begin with the gentle exercises of tightening the abdominal muscles, along with all the warm-up exercises except the squat. Stop exercises that increase your pain. As you become more active and have no pain, try the self-tests and do the exercises best suited for you.

If you need help, a physical therapist can guide your exercise program and your return to golf.

Applying these suggestions may help you resolve early symptoms before they progress, and you may prevent a major episode of back pain.

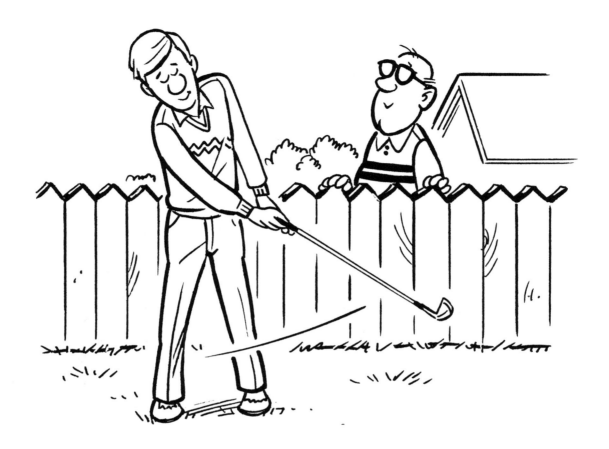

Your return to golf should progress gradually. When you are able to walk and exercise so that you can do the motions necessary for your golf swing, then you can begin to practice for your return.

Start practicing at home. Swing your club without hitting a ball to keep your swing more relaxed. Then concentrate your practice on putting and chipping. This will protect your back from too much rotation and it will probably help your score! Use only three balls to putt and chip so that you are forced to change your position frequently. When you are comfortable and feel confident, progress to a full swing.

Next, progress to hitting balls at a driving range. Follow the safe and smart routine of doing warm-up exercises. Work slowly at hitting a small bucket of balls, beginning your practice with chipping and gradually progressing to your full swing. Between shots, step away, line up your shot, and then return to addressing the ball. This will allow you to change your body position frequently.

Remember to take care of your back while driving, carrying your clubs, and getting into and out of your car. (See Chapter 5.)

When you are feeling strong and confident, return to play at the golf course.

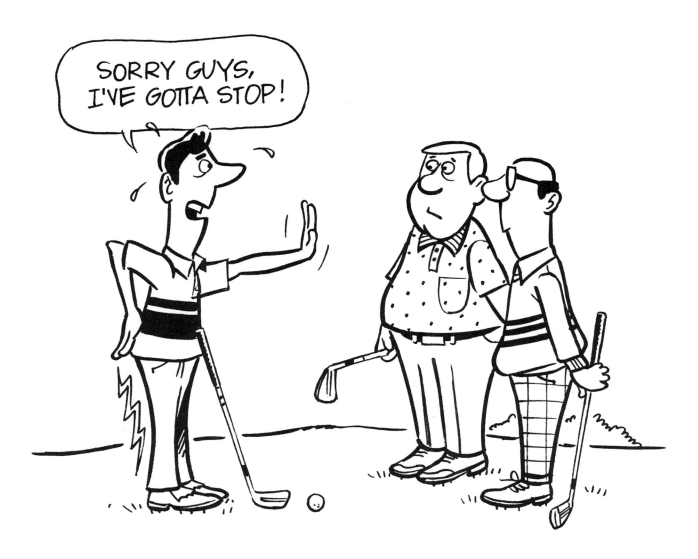

One question often asked is, "Should I continue to play golf or do other activities if I have pain?" You must be the judge of that by using the following guideline. If pain increases in intensity or spreads from back to thigh, calf, heel, or your upper back, then you **must stop** playing golf.

The first time you get back to golf, consider playing nine holes and be ready to stop playing if your symptoms reappear. Consider taking a penalty stroke if the ball is in a lie that will place undue stress on your back. You will find greater satisfaction by playing safely and preventing injury to your back.

113

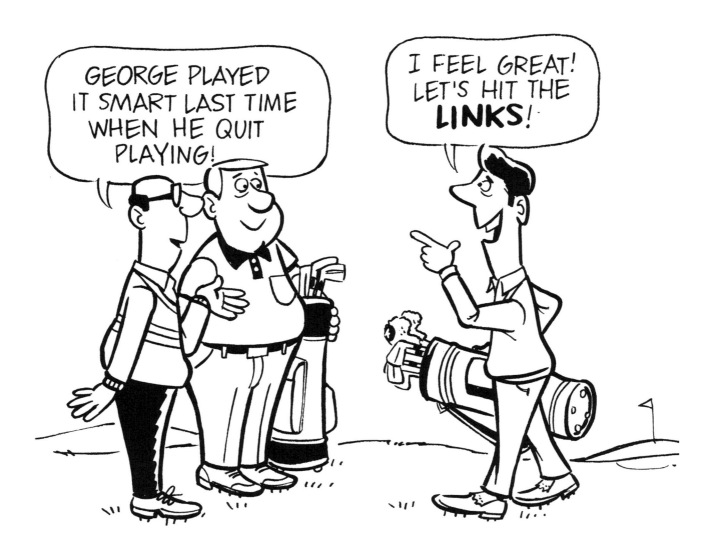

As you improve your fitness and gain control over pain, you may return to your level of play. With the information and modifications presented in this book, you can enjoy being on a golf course. You will be able to play for pleasure and relaxation or return to your level of competitive play.

Take care of your back so you can ***keep playing golf***!

SUGGESTED READINGS

Alcott, Amy, with Wade, Don. *Amy Alcott's Guide to Women's Golf.* New York: A Plume Book, published by the Penguin Group, 1993.

Coyne, John,. *Playing With the Pros: Golf Tips from the Senior Tour.* New York: Dutton, 1990.

The Fit Back: Prevention and Repair. Alexandria, VA: Time-Life Books.

Hay, Alex. *The Mechanics of Golf.* New York, St. Martin's Press, 1979.

"The Hidden Tips in Golf Injuries." *The Johns Hopkins Medical Letter.* Volume 2, Issue 5, July 1990.

Hogan, Ben. *Five Lessons: The Modern Fundamentals of Golf.* New York: A.S. Barnes and Company.

Irwin, Hale. *Play Better Golf with Hale Irwin.* London: Octopus Books Limited, 1980.

Jobe, Frank W. *Exercise Guide to Better Golf.* Inglewood, CA: Champion Press, 1994.

The Johns Hopkins Medical Handbook, prepared by the Editors of the Johns Hopkins Medical Letter "Health After Fifty." New York: Rebus, Inc. and Random House, Inc., 1992.

Kaskie, Shirli. *A Woman's Golf Game.* Chicago: Contemporary Books, Inc., 1982.

Kendall, Florence P.; McCreary, Elizabeth K.; and Provance, Patricia. *MUSCLES: Testing and Function.* Baltimore: Williams and Wilkins, 1993.

Kendall, Henry O.; Kendall, Florence P.; Boynton, Dorothy A. *Posture and Pain.* New York: Robert E. Krieger Publishing Co., Inc., 1977.

Lewis, Beverly. *Golf for Women.* Suffolk: Sackville Books, 1989.

Lopez, Nancy and Wade, Don. *Nancy Lopez's The Complete Golfer with Don Wade.* Chicago: Contemporary Books, Inc.

McLean, Jim, with Dennis, Larry. *Golf Digest's Book of Drills.* Connecticut: Golf Digest and New York: Pocket Books, 1990.

Nicklaus, Jack with Bowden, Ken. *Golf My Way.* Simon and Schuster, 1974.

Penick, Harvey with Shrake, Bud. *Harvey Penick's Little Red Book.* New York: Simon and Schuster, 1992.

Porterfield, James A, and DeRosa, Carl. *Mechanical Low Back Pain: Perspectives in Functional Anatomy.* Philadelphia: W.B. Saunders, 1991.

Root, Leon. *No More Aching Back.* New York: Villard Books, Random House, Inc,. 1990.

Saunders, H. Duane. *Golf and Back Pain: Does It Have To Hurt?* Minneapolis, MN: Saunders S'ports, 1992

Selby, Nancy. *My Aching Back!* The Spine Education Center's Back Care Book. Los Angeles: The Body Press, 1988.

Stover, Cornelius; McCarroll, John; and Mallon, William. *Feeling Up to Par.* Philadelphia: F.A. Davis Company, 1994.

White, Arthur H. and Anderson, Robert. *Conservative Care of Low Back Pain.* Baltimore: Williams and Wilkins, 1991.

White, Augustus A. *Your Aching Back, A Doctor's Guide to Relief.* New York: Simon & Schuster/ Fireside Books, 1990.

United States Golf Association, *Golf Rules in Pictures.* New York: The Putmam Publishing Group.

Videotape: *Good Golf for Bad Backs,* by Gary Winen, PhD and Jordan Grabel, M.D. Pro-Med Productions, Inc., 1993.

INDEX

Help Your Golfing Friends Take Care of Their Backs!

Order additional (or gift) copies of *Golfers, Take Care of Your Back*.
Check with your local bookstore, or order directly from us.

Ordered by: Name_____

Mailing Address_____

City_____

State_____Zip_____

Phone_____

To send order to different address than at left:

Ship to: Name_____

Mailing Address_____

City_____

State_____Zip_____

If this book is a gift, please print message below:

_____

_____

_____

Number of books _____ @ $16.50 (U.S.) each.................. Amount   _____
Handling charge for package sent to ONE address
$4 for up to 2 books plus $2 for each additional book....... Amount   _____

Handling charge for each additional address
$4 for up to two books plus $2 for each additional book... Amount   _____
                                                    Subtotal   _____
For books sent to New York residents, add 8% tax on the
cost of the books plus handling charges..........(8% tax in NY)   _____

For books sent to Maryland residents, add 5% tax on the
cost of the books plus handling charges..........(5% tax in MD)   _____

Additional Items Available:
Golf Bag Tag with Warm-Up Exercises @ $5.50 each......... Amount   _____
4 or more tags, $5.00 each..Amount   _____
Handling charge $2 for tags sent to one address................Amount   _____
(no additional handling charge for tags ordered with book)
taxes apply as above
                    TOTAL AMOUNT OF CHECK OR MONEY ORDER   _____

Make check or money order payable to: **Thistle Ridge Press**
                                        332 Bunn Hill Road
                                        Vestal, New York 13850
Do you have any comments or suggestions about the book?
We'd like to hear from you.